Past Caring

Audrey Jenkinson

Past Caring is dedicated to my beautiful
mother Audrey and my gentle father Eddie.
It is also dedicated to my big brother Haig and
my big sister Fiona. I am proud of the way you
have turned your lives around past caring.
Prouder still to be your sister.

Past Caring

Audrey Jenkinson

First published by Promenade Publishing 2003
Second Edition 2004

ISBN 09544233-6-4

Published by
Polperro Heritage Press
Clifton-upon-Teme
Worcestershire WR6 6EN

Cover design by Steve Bowgen

Printed by Orphans Press
Leominster HR6 8JT

Contents

Introduction

I don't know why it happened as it did. I don't know why they had to suffer as they did. I envied my friend whose dad collapsed midway through his Cuban cigar. I envied my neighbour. Her mother simply went to bed one night and never woke up. How lucky to just drop dead!

I know everyone must die. It is the how that is difficult to reconcile.

It was not so much my parents' deaths that scarred me but what they went through in their lives. If we could choose our deaths, oh joy! Choose our lives, what then? There would surely be a shortage of carers?

I had just turned twenty-four when my mother suffered a severe stroke. She had had a small one eight years previously. Fortunately, she recovered completely and I remained blissfully ignorant of the horrific damage a severe stroke could inflict. This time I was terrified. I moved back home from London, where I had been working as an actress. I was lost, out on a limb, didn't know what to do.

Whilst my friends were living the lives of twenty-somethings, excitedly buzzing with news of career, relationships and fashion, I found myself catapulted into a strange new world. The world of a family caring, as best we could, for a seriously ill loved one. It is a difficult world to put into words. I felt alone, often. How could I expect my friends to understand what was going on for me when it was so outwith their – my – ken?

Yes, we all have choices. Perhaps not about what events life deals us, but rather, what we choose to do about it. I moved back home. Twenty-four and terrified, a book was my saviour. *So They Tell Me: Encounter With Stroke* by Valerie Eaton Griffith, an account of the work she did, unpaid, purely as a neighbour, with the actress Patricia Neal, wife of the late Roald Dahl.

Patricia Neal had lost the power of her speech, as had my mother. Valerie's story, of her rehabilitation work with Pat, told with warmth and humour, kept me going. I now had a friend by my side, who had been there too, who *understood*.

Reading about other people in similar situations gave me a sense of not being quite so alone but somehow connected to the world. More importantly, it gave me a kind of hope, even in the bleakest days. Then – yet more bad news. We came to know that my father was once more suffering from cancer. He had had an operation to remove a tumour seven years previously. The cancer was back.

Witnessing what my parents endured and caring for them, along with my family, in the small ways we could, had an indelible effect on my being. I know this. *How* is more difficult to explain.

I saw things and heard things that haunt me still, I know. As I watched the life slowly ebb from my parents, so too did the life ebb from me. Like a pebble battered on the seashore I was eventually eroded, worn out. All this, *before* they died.

After they died, I know I hopped around like a little orphan lamb bleating every two minutes 'Life's so unfair.' I know I searched for reasons. Why do some souls seem to roll through life unscathed whilst others have to bear more than their fair share of tragedy? I couldn't understand it, tried to work it out.

Tony Garnet, a televison producer, once said to me, "Audrey, life is unfair. Once we accept that, it's easier." That made sense. Life is unfair. Why? Because it is. Some people have an easier time than others. Why? Because they do. Life is inexplicable. Things happen. We live the experience. We discover things about ourselves. We do our best. What else can we do?

To write a book like this was never in my plans. I could never have imagined that one day I would be sitting in strangers' living-rooms and offices across the country asking people about their life as a carer, as a past carer. But this is where I was led.

Nine and a half years ago, in the wake of the deaths of my mother and father, I went to a bookshop. I was searching. There were books on childbirth and menopause and 'Magical Living'. Books on health and wealth and finding Mr Right. Books on losing and gaining weight and how to have great sex. Books on general bereavement that advised the bereaved one to 'try to resume your normal life as soon as possible'.

But what if one's 'normal' life had been that of caring for the person who had died? What if one had given up more and more of one's own life to cope with the worsening illness and demands of caring for another? There was nothing on how to face the challenge of filling the void. Where to begin? After years of caring, what do you do with freedom?

It really bothered me that there was no book on this subject. A seed was planted. As an actress I needed a creative way to try to make sense of my parents suffering. My father was a writer. I had looked for a book that didn't exist. So why didn't I write one?

The good news ... here's the book.

The bad news ... forget nine and a half weeks; it took me nine and a half years.

Although the *idea* of the book possessed me, I was scared. Scared I couldn't do it. Years of caring had filled my once carefree being with endless doubt, confusion. As a child, I believed anything was possible. As a young adult I still believed it. Then came the years of my parents' illness, the juggling of caring and career, the exhaustion, the panic attacks, the loss of joy, the guilt, the fear. The constant terror inside, the not knowing, what will today bring?

I woke up one morning to find my once bubbly pool of confidence had evaporated.

I no longer had any sense of self. It was as if someone had gutted my fleshy centre and left just a bony shell. I could function and look fairly normal from the outside but the inside was empty. It was hard to remember that I was once the girl from Leith who had dreamt of going to London and getting a part on television.

Self-esteem plummeted. I trailed along Harley Street desperate for plastic surgery because I believed myself so incredibly ugly. "Don't worry, we can fix you," said cheery consultants. I was ready to sign up for anything, I was willing to risk everything such was my lack of self-love. (Thankfully, I was rescued by a dear friend, though not before I had a small bump filed down on my nose. It's now worse!) I have nothing against plastic surgery, but I believe the decision to go ahead with it should be made from a solid perspective. The thought that I almost signed up to have my entire face restructured now amazes me.

This incredible loss of confidence is something I have struggled with over the years since my parents died. If they had just dropped dead one fine day, would that have affected my being in such a way? I cannot say. All I know is that the years of caring took their toll as they did.

The idea of this book stayed with me but I couldn't see the way ahead.

Then, suddenly, after years of self-destructing with grief, living in chaos and craziness, I found a way. Not alone, *but with the help of others.*

I sought out human beings who had cared for other human beings twenty-four hours a day for no pay, for nothing but love. People who had seen terrible things yet stood firm in the face of their own fear to offer what comfort they could to a dying loved one.

I interviewed Christians, Quakers, Hindus and heathens. I spoke to those who had lost faith and those who had found faith. I interviewed children who had cared for parents and parents who had cared for children. I talked to husbands that cared for wives, and wives husbands. I met with men and women who happily shared their stories in a bid to help other men and women like them. And with each story I heard, I came to know more the tremendous scope of the human spirit and its extraordinary ability to survive the most profound tragedies, to not only survive but transform the darkest days even, into a dazzling new dawn.

I came to know that in past caring there is no right or wrong. That what is important is to honour our pain, sit with it, live with it. Trust that it will lead us to a new place.

Words seem inadequate to capture the depth of emotion that is at the core of each individual's experience. Feelings are to be felt, lived. Only then do words come. And in words there is a chance to share experiences, to know that you are not alone.

Past Caring is a sharing of stories. They are personal stories that have been generously told to me. My hope is that they will in some way touch and inspire those who read them. This book was born from a wish to give something back. It is a thank you to Valerie Eaton Griffith who took time to document her story and make a difference in my life.

With love, Audrey.

Care Fact

There are over seven million informal carers in the UK today.

Over seven million people currently looking after an ill relative or friend at home.

Seven million.

That's more than the entire population of Scotland, almost one thousand, seven hundred and seventy-seven packed jumbo jets; enough people to fill Ibrox 117 times and if you laid seven million people end to end (average height 5'7") you would cover a distance of seven and a half thousand miles. That's like walking half-way across the world, half-way from Scotland to Australia. Phew, that's a lot of worn out soles.

Some day, over seven million souls will be past caring. Unbelievably no book has ever been written on the subject of what life is like for people past caring.

Care Fact

Most carers and past carers feel isolated and alone. If you feel isolated and alone, here's the good news …

There are six million, nine hundred and ninety-nine thousand, nine hundred and ninety-nine human beings out there who probably feel just like you.

"Every time I drive past a hospital, I think of all the ill people inside that building. I think of how many of them will be going home today, tomorrow. And I think of all the people who love them, who become carers overnight."

Mary Parsons,
a sole carer for both parents for thirty years.

Part 1

MY STORY

Caring is not always, but was in my case, a family affair. There were many players in the caring act. My Dad, brother, sister, uncles, aunts, cousins, good neighbours and friends of my parents' united in help.

If I say too little about the stories of my brother, who remained at home and was, in essence, the main carer for my mother after my father died ... or my sister, who was married with three young children of her own to care for, it is because I care about my brother and sister not too little but too much. It is up to them, if they choose, to tell their stories. I thank them for their understanding of my need to tell my story.

Memory – Sixteen years old

I am excited, terribly. I am away from home for a whole summer. I am staying in Stirling, a mere hour from Edinburgh. But such is the adventure, I could be on the moon!

I am in The Scottish Youth Theatre. Yippee! I got picked, I'm in, I'm in Stirling. There are around fifty of us, aspiring thespians, aged between fourteen and eighteen. We are loud and giggly and greet each other with great big hugs, darling. We bounce around Stirling University campus like a litter of eager puppies discovering their new-found freedom. There's lots of instant bonding, lots of secrets shared, betrayed, lots of friendships forged, broken. There are confessions of undying love or lust during midnight games of truth or dare.

By day there are workshops with famous and not-so-famous directors, there is singing and dancing and drum-banging, there is nail-biting news of casting. There is rehearsal, rehearsal, rehearsal, punctuated by tears, laughter and tantrums. Our efforts will cumulate in a grand production at the end of the summer. The audience will consist primarily of beaming parents.

Our production this year is named *Sun Circle* and is some kind of complicated tale about ancient Druids. It is the only sun to grace Stirling that summer. Typically the days are soaking wet but nothing can dampen my spirits. My greatest wish is to be a professional actress. I am here, in Stirling, where magical things may happen. The summer stretches endlessly ahead.

I call home. My brother answers. I am bursting with news, chatting on. He listens patiently, then:

"Hang on, I'll get Dad."

There is something in his voice. What?

"Hi, Turkey." (I still have no idea why my Dad called me Turkey but he called me it when I was wee and it stuck.) "How're you?"

"Great."

Dad's voice sounds strange.

" I've bad news."

My stomach flips.

"Mum's in hospital. But she's fine."

"What happened?"

I hear my voice tremble.

"She's fine now, okay, don't worry …"

"What happened?"

"We found her unconscious on the kitchen floor. She's had a wee stroke."

"What's a stroke?"

It was against the odds. Out of the norm. "Unlucky, very". I found out, later, strokes were usually the curse of people in their sixties, seventies, eighties, but rarely in their forties.

Nobody could really explain why. It was "one of those things".

I wanted to return home, but my father said, stay, stay, do your acting, mum wants that too, you stay in Stirling. He reassured me she was fine, just a tiny slurring of her speech, the doctors thought that would sort itself out, yes, she'd be home soon, yes, I could speak to her then, yes, yes he promised to call the Youth Theatre office if anything changed.

I hung up the phone. Suddenly *Sun Circle* didn't seem so important. Excitement replaced by overwhelming fear.

I am sixteen years old. My powerful, vivacious mum has been struck down, with no warning, by something called a stroke. Yesterday the world was a safe place. Today it is a scary place. Strokes at forty-eight. *Sun Circle* shattered.

In a way, I was lucky. At sixteen, it was my first encounter with a loved one being ill. I'd had relatives who had died but that was different. They just died. Or so it seemed to me as a child.

My Grandma, who had lived with us, had died of a heart-attack when I was five years old. I couldn't remember her being ill. It seemed she was there one minute, gone the next. I was so disappointed because I had been due to start school and was desperate to show Grandma my spanking new school uniform. How inconsiderate, to leave before I could parade my snazzy outfit! I was told that Grandma was now in heaven and yes, she would still be able to see me in my new school uniform from 'a cloud'. In bed, late at night, I used to talk to her, plead with her, to come down, just one last time to see me. It would be our secret. I used to get up and peer out of my bedroom window, fully expecting her to be there, outside in the darkness, waiting. I couldn't understand it – surely she would come back for me?

After Grandma died, Mum was quick to upset. I hated seeing my mummy upset. I would take her hand and tell her that had I been a nurse Grandma wouldn't have died. I would tell her that if she, Mummy, ever got ill, she needn't worry because I would be a big grown-up nurse and I wouldn't let her die.

When I was eleven, my dear Uncle Donald died of a heart attack. He went to the hospital and died within twenty-four hours.

So at sixteen, I was in a sense, sheltered from, if not death, illness.

At school, I had a casual friend whose Dad died of cancer. I only ever once went to her house. I remember her father sitting by a blazing fire, though it was a sweltering day. He was wearing an orange crocheted cap and had a bashed-in face like a skull. I was both frightened and fascinated. Trisha's weary mum handed us two blue plastic cups of orange juice and told us "go play in the garden, and don't make too much noise, mind". I was glad to get outside. We sat on the warm grass sipping our orange juice.

"How did your Dad get cancer?"

"Dunno."

"How long has he had it?"

"Ages."

"Will he die?"

"Think so."

"When?"

"Dunno. C'mon, let's play hide n'seek."

Naïve shrieks of hide n'seek whilst, inside, only feet away, a man, a father, sat dying. In our playing, soon forgotten.

Memory – Seventeen years old

I am awakened in the middle of the night by blood-curling screams. In a daze, I leap from my bed and race into my parents' bedroom. My mum is writhing in agony, screaming like a banshee, sweat pouring from her. I ask, "what's wrong Mum, what's wrong?" But she is screaming so she cannot speak. Dad is phoning a doctor. I think my Mum is surely about to die.

X-rays reveal Mum has broken ribs. Unbeknown to us, she had fallen earlier that evening onto the stone fireplace. The stroke has left her with a small limp in her right leg. She is not as steady as she used to be.

As a milky-dawn breaks, I lie awake, unable to sleep. My heart is pounding so hard and I can't stop my body from doing the St Vitas' dance. Is this what adults call 'nerves'?

Mum is sore for weeks. By day, I am at school, Dad at work, brother at university, sister at teacher training. Various aunts, uncles and good neighbours keep an eye on her. For nights afterward, I doze fitfully, listening out for strange sounds of distress, ready to dash through any moment, as if a young mother listening out for a newborn babe.

Memory – Nineteen years old

I am on a jumbo jet crossing the giant pond, heading home to Scotland.

I have been away for a whole summer, to a place much more exciting than Stirling. My suitcase is crammed with nick-knacks of New York and Traverse City, Michigan. Pressies for everyone. For myself, a summer of fond memories that I replay again and again.

I have spent most of the summer in Traverse City, a small, pleasant holiday town on the shore of Lake Michigan, full of colourful wooden houses with verandahs. I have survived a slave-driven season as an 'apprentice' doing summer stock theatre. I have performed countless children's shows for an army of uncontrollable North American teenies. I arranged this trip myself, to visit America, with a view to developing my 'art'. My claim to fame is having been a Magic Mouse and a runaway hen!

At the invitation of a fellow apprentice, I have spent the last ten days in New York, a guest of her wealthy family. I have been chauffeured up and down Park Avenue in a limousine, I have seen shows on Broadway, I have sipped tea at the Plaza. I have stood at the top of the world, gazing up at the stars. New York, city of dreams, is intoxicating. I am an actress, almost. Upon my return to Scotland, I will enter my second year at drama school and … who knows?

When the cab draws up, I see Mum waving from the window. I feel a surge of joy. The joy of being home, of being cared for. My Mum has been watching out for me. Smiling, she comes down the path. Apart from the limp, she has completely recovered from the stroke. We hug and kiss, she says, "you look well", I say, "you too Mum", but the truth is she looks tired.

We make straight for the kitchen. The kettle is already boiling. I tell her that Americans make terrible tea. She laughs, then turns serious.

"I need to tell you something. Dad's not been well."

… fear seeping into my guts …

"What's happened?

"… cancer."

No! Cancer is what happens to other people's dads.

"They got the tumour."

"Why didn't you tell me?"

My voice is shaking …

"We didn't want to worry you Audrey. He's okay, he's okay …"

As if on cue, my Dad is suddenly standing in the doorway.

"See, I'm okay. I'm okay," he says gently, his eyes glistening.

My strong Dad, looking as if some cannibal has removed half his fleshy face. My Dad, who goes to work each day in a suit and is the sports editor of our local evening newspaper, who has his photo in the paper presenting one cup or another to somebody or another. My Dad, he of the dry wit and cheeky grin, who loves a wee dram and a flutter on the greyhounds, who is a fair man, a good man, my Dad, who once scooped me out of a thick bed of nettles when I fell off the wall … How could he get …?

I choke back tears. I don't want to upset him. I hug him tight. He's so thin.

"Oh Dad, Dad …"

"I'm okay. I'm okay," he repeats again and again as mum pours us all a nice strong cup of tea.

I cry when I am alone. I cry for my brave Dad who, I learn, has endured two operations, severe septicaemia and who now has a bag instead of a bowel. "A lucky bag," I had laughed. Sometimes I laugh when I am afraid. Afraid of what might happen next.

Memory – Twenty two years old

I have graduated from drama school. I am an actress! I am so chuffed to be cast in a theatre show, a comedy called *Wedding Fever*. Directed by Scottish icon, Jimmy Logan, I am playing the daughter of a die-hard Rangers supporter who wishes to marry her sweetheart, Dennis, the son of a fanatical Celtic supporter. With the innocence of youth, we can't see what our families are making such a fuss about. So we decide to invite the two families to meet and all hell breaks loose.

We have been playing to packed houses at the King's Theatre, Glasgow. Tonight my parents are in the audience. I am nervous, extremely. I pray it goes well. It does. The roars of laughter come thick and fast.

Afterwards, I rush out to meet my parents. My Mum is sitting in the foyer, gripping her forehead. She has been having terrible headaches recently, like a vice squeezing her brain. When she sees me she smiles, "well done darling". Anxiety floods my being. I wish these awful headaches would go away.

Some days she is well. Oh joy, relief. We go out, up the town, have lunch in Jenners. Other days are cursed. Headaches, dizziness, nausea. Painkillers don't make a difference. Doctors don't know what to do. I try to help but I am helpless. I massage her head, brush her hair, nothing eases it. Seeing her in pain makes me feel sick of heart. I wish these headaches would leave us all in peace. Please God.

Memory – Twenty-three years old

I have been in the Big Smoke for two whole days and I am hooked. I love the hustle bustle, the big red buses, trains that whizz underground, the neon lights that buzz night and day around the theatres on Shaftesbury Avenue.

I have found a pleasant room in a Victorian terraced house. I have enrolled at the Actors Centre. I have a London agent. I feel like life is opening up, full of possibilities.

I call home from a payphone in Piccadilly Circus.

"Hi, Dad, it's me."

Dad is at home now having taken early retirement due to ill-health.

"I love London, Dad. There's so much to do."

"That's good."

We chat for a bit. When I ask to speak to Mum he tells me she is in bed. He says she has had a little 'mini-turn', just for a few seconds she lost consciousness, but then was fine, apparently the doctor says it is something called a transient ischemic attack. Apparently that kind of thing sometimes happens to people who have had strokes. Dad assures me she's okay and in bed, resting. I say to tell her I called and I'll call later.

I hang up the phone, utterly deflated. How serious is it? Should I get on the train and go home? What if I get on the train and go home and she's completely fine? What if I don't get on the train and go home and she's not fine? What if she dies? I stand in the middle of Piccadilly Circus, lost.

Memory – Twenty-four years old

The noise in the Tewkesbury theatre is tumultuous as cries of "He's behind you, *he's behind you*" grow more desperate. We, the actors, deliberately look the other way, as the young audience leap up and down, frantically pointing. It's Panto season. Cinderella. I am dressed in nothing more than a shiny blue tunic and flesh-coloured tights, wishing I had done heaps more exercise before baring my thighs in public. It is a gruelling schedule. We perform two hectic shows a day, lots of smiling, singing, dancing, zany high-energy fun.

After a slow start in London, life is going well. I have played a damsel in distress in a new children's series, then a tarty barmaid in a BBC play, then straight to Panto through January 12th, then … who knows?

Tomorrow is Christmas day, a day off. I am spending the day with my new boyfriend at his wee Wiltshire cottage. His parents are staying over, his mum has kindly offered to cook Christmas dinner. There will be champagne and chocolates. There will be a long walk in the countryside, then lazing before the fire like a contented walrus, watching *The Wizard of Oz* … the old thigh-exercises can wait 'til next year.

Christmas morning and I revel in bed, enjoying the lie-in. At 11am, I call home to say Happy Christmas. My Dad tells me that Mum has suffered a severe stroke. It happened after breakfast the day before.

"Let me talk to her."

"She can't speak …" My Dad sounds shocked, like he can't believe it. *I can't believe it.*

"But she must be able to say something."

"Nothing …"

No! Please no …

"Write things down?"

"She can't understand letters. The doctor says they will look like a foreign language to her. The clot has wiped out the communication part of the brain. And …"

I can't breathe.

"… she's paralysed down one side."

As neighbours file into the house, having been invited for Christmas drinks, I hide up stairs, lying on the bed, with the curtains closed. I imagine my spirited chatty Mum lying paralysed, unable to speak. It is unimaginable. Laughter and cheery chatter drift upstairs, as I weep. I go for a walk alone. I notice nothing but the sick, twisted feeling in my guts. The beautifully prepared dinner lies untouched on my plate. At night, I turn away from my boyfriend. *Paralysed, unable to speak.* I don't know how Mum will get through it; how any of us will get through it, this nightmare.

The pantomime is booked up. I don't have an understudy. The show goes on. I will visit Mum on New Year's Eve.

I am like a wound-up toy, one more turn and I will snap, break. Weight falls off me – who needs exercise? The new Tense Nervous Wonder-Diet. Amazing, shed a stone in a week. I don't want sex, don't want to be touched, held. Shut the world out. It takes every ounce of concentration to get through each performance. The heavy pantomime make-up is a perfect mask, as I laugh and joke with the audience then rush back-stage to phone home.

We had planned a romantic New Year at a London party. Instead my boyfriend chauffeured me to Heathrow. He had said he'd come to Scotland, but I said no, I want to go home alone. I also wanted to protect a private and proud woman, now utterly helpless.

I was both desperate and terrified to see Mum. Terrified of what I was about to see.

Up-close, there was no escaping the horrific damage done by the stroke. There, lying in the bed, was my beautiful Mum, now sporting the haunted look of a woman way older than her fifty-five years.

My Mum … who, as a child had asked her father if she could attend elocution lessons to learn how to 'speak nicely', who loved to write and recite poetry, who could deliver all twenty-three verses of Tam o' Shanter by heart, who loved a good natter with friends, who would sing songs with me on her knee, us watching Bill and Ben and Camberwick Green, my Mum, who loved to dance and dance and laugh at our neighbourhood New Year soirees.

My Mum … there before me, floppy right side propped up by pillows, one eye drooping as if drunk or drugged, one hand curled tightly like a claw, a mouth cruelly twisted, dribbling saliva … nothing could have prepared me for this.

I wanted to run out the room, shout stop, re-wind, start again, like they do in Hollywood movies. Life does not afford the luxury.

I placed a bunch of yellow carnations on the bedside table and hugged her, kissed her. Oh Mum, oh Mum, I whispered. She was sobbing, throaty staccato gulps, like an erratic machine gun. She tried to speak but only deep growling sounds came out. Panic danced in her wild eyes. The growling increased to a demented howl, a roar, like that of a wounded animal. I stood, helpless. All I could do was hold her and whisper I love you, Mum, I love you, shhh, shhh, it's okay, it's okay … But I knew it wasn't okay, it was very much not okay, never would be okay again. The nightmare was now reality.

On 13 January, I bade farewell to Cinderella and flew home. I arrived armed with umpteen books on strokes and their prevention (a bit like bolting the stable door you might say!) Stroke patients need to be treated like 'normal'. It was impossible to predict how well stroke victims would recover, but it was important to remain positive. Stroke victims should not be ignored, patronised or parked in front of a telly all day. Stroke victims, like anyone, need 'stimulation'.

I arrived home like a warrior going into battle. The battle of winning against an enemy called stroke. I became a how-to daughter; how to lower cholesterol, how to give up smoking, how to lower blood pressure … a girl on a mission. Oat bran was sprinkled liberally on cereal (Mum would screw up her face in disgust); cigarettes were hidden out of sight; oranges replaced chocolate.

The plan was that I would stay at home for a few weeks, then return south. That was the plan. But in the words of Rabbie B, 'the best laid schemes o'mice and men gang aft agley'.

This period of time, the months after my mother was struck down by her second stroke, was one of the toughest, most testing times of my life. I was at home for five months.

It was not just the physical care of my Mum, the assisting with washing and dressing and feeding, but the emotional care. My Mum was an inspiration to us, the way she fiercely fought to get well. She always had a stubborn streak, and this now served her. Refusing to be defeated she would insist on getting out of bed each day and getting washed and dressed no matter how daunting the thought. (Her valiant efforts were rewarded when some strength came back in her right leg.)

However, during the course of the day and night, several times or more, it would seem that the shock of what had happened would hit her afresh and her brave spirit would simply dissolve in overwhelming despair. In these moments she would collapse, cry and cry and cry as though her heart was breaking. I have never seen such tears. I would cuddle her and whisper soothing words of encouragement trying to be strong, trying to be positive, though my own heart was breaking.

How do you communicate with someone who cannot speak, who cannot write things down, who cannot read, who has no understanding whatsoever of the written word?

It was at times like these that I wished I had paid more attention in the dreaded mime classes at drama school!

Mum knew exactly what she wanted to say only she could not connect the thought to formulate a word. She knew everything that was going on around her, understood everything that was said to her. Imagine, for a second, that you knew what you wanted to say but no matter how hard you tried, no words came out of your mouth. Imagine the sheer frustration.

Our days were filled with asking Mum hundreds of questions to which she would shake or nod her head. Are you in pain? Is it about me? You? Dad? Haig? Fiona? The dog? Does it hurt? Is it about food? Is it about a place? Is it about … on and on, question upon question, like a game of charades, except no-one can yell the answer when one says, I give up. If we were way off the subject matter Mum would get visibly agitated, her eyes flashing with annoyance, her good left fist making circles in the air. At the sight of this our questions would get increasingly more desperate, until frustration won out and the episode would end with us both in tears. Count to ten, cuddle and start all over again. The prison walls were sturdy but we would keep trying to break through them.

I recall one time when I had spent hours – *hours* – trying to figure out what Mum wanted to know. I had asked so many questions it sounded like I had digested an encyclopaedia. Mum was beside herself. I finally struck gold – Mum wanted to know *what day it was*. I told her, "it's Tuesday Mum, Tuesday." She nodded and lay back, exhausted, delighted, like a woman who had just conquered Everest.

In addition to caring for Mum, my Dad and brother (who had his own business) kept everything ticking over at home, went shopping and picked up prescriptions. My Dad would cook. I was in charge of speech therapy and physio. (Mum was given an hour a week at our local hospital, but could not attend for the first few weeks as she wasn't well enough. I think this kind of service, one hour a week, is hopeless for stroke patients with severe speech problems.)

Mum had lost the feeling down one side of her face. She had lost the ability to imitate a simple sound. If I sat in front of her and made a vowel sound "Ah" or a consonant sound "Mmm", and asked her to copy me, she would be completely lost. Even if we used a mirror, she simply could not begin to arrange her mouth in the correct position to make the sound. What I discovered, almost by accident, was that if I linked the sound to an obvious image, the image or picture in Mum's head triggered the sound without her thinking too hard about it. I would say okay Mum, imagine you're in the middle of the sea and you're a big hungry fish and you want to gobble up as many of the little fishes as you can so you open your mouth really really wide and you say "Ah". "Ah" Mum would repeat. Then I might say okay, you're really starving and Dad's just put down a delicious meal and you go "Mmmm". I would exaggerate the sound, make the images funny or silly, anything to entertain her. We did those sounds, simple sounds over and over and over and over again, day in, day out.

It was hard work and required the utmost concentration. Mum would tire quickly. We found it was best to do it in regular shorter bursts rather than attempt a big session. We discovered that Mum could often fill in the one last word of a nursery rhyme if I sung it out loud. We learned that the singing part of the brain was in a different sphere to the speaking. We did arm exercises and hand exercises. A millimetre of movement was a victory. The tiniest of a pure sound was a triumph.

The days were relieved by visits from aunts, uncles, friends, neighbours bearing well-meaning but often cholesterol-laden gifts. Mum would welcome this distraction, tea would be made, chairs pulled up around the fire.

After the initial confusion about where folk should direct their gaze – should they look to Mum and say how are you? – knowing she could not reply, or should they say to us – How is she doing? as if Mum was not there, we settled on the former. We believed it best for Mum to be treated as 'normal', even if we were her voice, answering back like some trite ventriloquist. Woe betide if we got it wrong (often!), Mum would glare, we would hurriedly invent a new possibility. Of course, then Mum would want to ask the visitors questions and so the guessing game went on, back and forth, ping-pong-ping, utterly exhausting but necessary.

My big sister and her husband were regular visitors with their three young children. It was amazing to watch the children, aged three, five and seven interact with Mum. They were sensitive and kind and were not afraid. My sister had done an excellent job explaining to them what had happened, and they carried on as usual, accepting the change in their simple child-like way. Sometimes they giggled at Mum's bleating sounds, and we would tell them that was how they had sounded before they could speak, just a lot of gurgly incoherent sounds. This would make them giggle even more. They would quite happily climb up on the sofa and install themselves next to their grandma and try to guess what she was trying to say too. Only one cousin didn't bring his children to see my Mum. He said he didn't want to scare them. My view is that it was not his children who may be scared, but himself.

Being face to face with illness is scary. You cannot help but imagine yourself in that position. I was amazed what could happen to human beings and still they live. I was scared Mum would take another stroke and die, or perhaps worse, take another stroke and survive?

Each milky dawn brought both terror and hope. Hope because Mum had survived another day, terror because another stroke may take her today. This fear, this unbearable tension was exhausting to the nervous system. It drained me to the core. I am sure too, my brother and Dad. It was like being suspended on a tightrope, no safety net, limbo-land. One time, as Dad and I sat having a late night cup of tea, he confided: "Each day I feel like I'm treading water, treading water really hard just to keep afloat."

Day and night merged into one, weeks mashed together in a blur. I said hello to my ribcage for the first time in years. I looked like I had had liposuction on my cheeks. My whole body was shrinking, everything caving in. Even my once bubbly voice sounded thin and feeble. Nights of broken sleep painted purple half-moons under each eye. Any auditions going for ghost films?

My life as an actress seemed a lifetime away. Friends would ring up with news of what they were up to, auditions, parts in plays. What party they went to where, what they were wearing, not wearing, who they were sleeping with, not sleeping with, whom they would like to. I loved and hated them. I envied their fortunes and frivolous talk. I would lie on the floor, phone in hand, giving monosyllabic answers, paralysed by fatigue. As my friends set off for a ritzy night on the town, I would crawl into bed and curl up with my book

Encounter With Stroke. Valerie Eaton Griffith gave me comfort. She threw me a lifeline that I grasped tightly. She saved me. .

My original plan of being home for three weeks seemed laughable. I did and did not want to leave. Mum's progress was painstakingly slow, but progress nonetheless. She would roll her eyes to the heavens when I took out the homegrown 'speak-easy' box. We would do different sounds, Mum would repeat them after me, I would ask her to do one on her own and she was lost. I discovered patience. I discovered how to persevere in the face of no result, when effort seemed futile. This was far tougher than any acting work.

My relationship did not survive. I had not one ounce of energy to give to it. Once, when I went to visit my boyfriend, with the best of intentions, he had planned a weekend of 'fun things to do'. "But I planned to stay in bed for the weekend", I moaned. He lit up but was soon disappointed. I meant to stay in bed to sleep. And sleep. And sleep.

We split up. It wasn't his fault. I was narky and couldn't communicate, at a loss to articulate how I felt. (I have since learned that when we are in the middle of a trauma we are not so able to express ourselves. We are too busy dealing with it, getting through. Only once we are safely on the other side and have some distance from it may we begin to have some understanding of the way we were affected by it.)

All the hard work paid off one glorious day when Mum said her first word. I was hiding them behind my back, I didn't want her to have one, she wanted one, was desperate. Garbled, but yes, a single word – "*Cid-urr-ette*". It popped out, uninvited. Mum looked shocked, twizzled round as if to say "Who said that?" I flung my arms around her, ecstatic. Yes, Yes, You, You said it Mum, you said *cigarette*. She giggled, cried and lit up.

In late May, I returned to London. Late spring, pink and white blossom enveloping Hampstead Heath. It was strange, starting over, finding a room, moving my stuff there to here. Almost five months unemployed, I felt so 'out' of the acting scene. I knew how easily actors are forgotten, how quickly faces blend into each other as the powers that be simply call someone else, oh she's not around, okay, next. I was ambitious, eager to get acting work. Yet I didn't want to abandon the speech work and, when needed, be there to boost Mum's morale. Like Pooh Bear I needed a plan. Eureka! I would spend two weeks in London, two weeks in Edinburgh, two weeks in London, two weeks in Edinburgh and so on …

I also wanted to be in Edinburgh simply to *be* with Mum. Knowing another stroke could steal her away forever, gnawing need overtook me, a need to make the most of our time together or rather what was left of it. So every two weeks, I had the tawdry but life-enhancing experience of travelling on the overnight bus between London and Edinburgh.

The summer sent bluer skies, Mum would be well enough to go to lunch, the hairdresser, Princes Street Gardens. Dad or my brother (who did an amazing job of running his own business *and* caring for Mum), would take her runs in the car, down the Borders, over to Fife. There were laughs. There were tears. There were days when we got ratty with each other – Mum would then tell me to "fly away home…" "But Mum, I am home …" Mum would purse her lips, a lop-sided grin *yoo shud op*. Amidst the sorrow of the stroke, we could laugh again.

A seesaw existence between London and Scotland proved tiring. I was a canoeist with a foot in each canoe paddling upstream in danger of splitting in two. Dating men was hard. Unlike Julie Andrews, my 'Getting To Know You' never quite zipped along with any momentum. Rather it got stuck on bar one. If I did have coffee or dinner with someone I might not be able to see them again for ages. I could see them thinking, oh yeh, this is the brush off, she's not interested, yeh, see you in three weeks, maybe.

And then there was the effort. The effort of explaining. What had happened, what had happened before that and that and that and. Dates were supposed to be fun, uplifting, playful. Dates were not supposed to leave some poor unsuspecting soul reaching for the razor blades. Dating seemed like Sisyphus and his rock, such a mammoth effort. Far easier to prevaricate in public and worry home alone.

Since my parents fell ill, anxiety had taken root in my being. I had become a worrier. What about Dad, would his cancer come back? What about Mum? How was she doing? Would she get better? What if something else happened? This anxiety took root. Began to grow. Day by day.

Over time, Mum's speech slowly improved, minuscule breakthroughs, until she could say more single words and could understand some written words. She became adept at working with her left hand and took to following my father around in 'her' kitchen, much to our joy and his annoyance, rearranging things to her liking as he tried to cook. She would insist, to our trepidation, on making pots of tea, pouring the scalding water with her left hand. So, she began, in ways, to care for us again. She was still our mother, lest we forget. Though her speech had been snatched so cruelly she had a good pair of lungs and knew how to use them. If displeased she roared. She was still 'the boss'.

This feisty determination gave her the courage to fight. With her left hand, she practised fastening buttons and brushing her teeth and copying the letters of the alphabet, utterly concentrated, twisting the pencil this way and that for hours. My most treasured possession is a birthday card I received for my twenty-fifth birthday – it is a child-like scrawl but it is my name all right – 'To Dear Audrey, Love, Mum xxx'.

Memory – Twenty-five years old

After months of unemployment I am cast in an outdoor theatre show, performing against the backdrop of the stunning Forth Rail Bridge. I am staying at home. Mum has not been well. My brother is working all hours. All my energy has been taken up with the show. I am aware that Dad has a lot to contend with. I am in a show. I can't do any more. I feel bad. Mum and Dad don't see the show. I feel sad.

Memory – Twenty-five years old

I am in London, chatting on the phone to my best friend Joanna, laughing, gossiping about nothing in particular. She has known me since I was fifteen. I suddenly hear myself saying "I can't remember, I can't remember my Mum's voice, I can't remember what it sounds like, oh God, why can I not remember, I just can't, I can't remember her voice", and then I am howling, in danger of bursting poor Joanna's eardrums as she says, I'm coming over.

Memory – Twenty-six years old

I am astride an enormous racehorse on the magnificent Berkshire Downs. An icy March breeze numbs my fingers, face, toes, actually *everything*. On 'Action!' I walk the horse directly toward the camera. He strides out, powerful, graceful, the wind wildly blowing his mane. I grip the reins and pray he doesn't tipple that I am only a learner, whisk me off for a joyride, a high-speed break-necking spin. He behaves perfectly. I dismount and plant a thank-you kiss on his neck before my shivering body is encased in a giant BBC parka and someone thrusts a polystyrene cup of tea in my frozen hands. I see Susannah York and David McCallum grinning from the comfort of a cosy Landrover. Who said filming was glamorous?

Just turned twenty-six and a dream come true. I have worked hard for this dream. I have made a hundred phone calls, written a thousand letters. I have taken up residence outside the BBC handing my photo and CV to unsuspecting producers. I have risked rejection after rejection and now a tiny seed has taken root. For the BBC I am playing a rough'n'tumble stable-girl named Mo, who dreams of being a champion jockey. For real, I am Audrey Jenkinson from Edinburgh who long ago dreamt of playing a stable-girl … actually, *anything* … for the BBC. This is the bees-knees. Since forever I have been pony-mad and now I get to ride racehorses for a whole nine months? A nine-month contract! It is the first week of March. I have been filming since 14 January. Seven and a half months still to go. Bliss.

I am renting a room in a beautiful thatched cottage in the village of Compton. The owners are a lovely easy-going arty-farty family. We are immediately friends.

That night after filming, I call home as usual. Only this night my brother tells me Dad is in bed with 'stomach pains'. My heart skips.

"Do they think it's his … old problem?" I say, scared to say the dreaded 'C' word.

"No," says my brother. "The doctor thinks it's gastro-enteritis."

It wasn't gastro-enteritis. I flew home. For ten whole days my Dad lay in his bed and he couldn't eat and he couldn't drink and his stomach furiously spat and gurgled and groaned and still the doctors said, "Don't worry, it's just a bug."

I know. I was there in the room. I saw everything.

He was in terrific pain. He was brave, but also afraid. He grew weaker and vomited blood. The doctors came and shook their heads and said, "It's a bad bug." Finally, after ten terrible days and nights, they admitted him to hospital.

They did not one, but two operations, cut out the cancer, hooked him to a ventilator in intensive care. I didn't want to leave him. The dream-job now an ordeal to get through.

Sadly, my Dad never got out of intensive care, but he battled with every ounce of his being and survived for an amazing ten weeks. He defied medical opinion. (Against all the odds he would eventually breathe on his own, unaided.) We lurched from hope to no hope and hope once more. We didn't know whether to say 'Goodbye' or 'C'mon Dad, you can do it!' This terrible not knowing ... unexpected dips and peaks, a sickening roller-coaster, now racing, now reversing. We dealt with this with tears and hysterics and black humour. Twice, thrice a day we'd wait outside the IC ward, wait whilst they 'got him ready' and my brother and I, twitching with nervy laughter, would occupy ourselves speculating futures. "Bet that guy in the unit next to Dad will be gone, he was mustard colour, and the woman with the bald head and tattoo definitely gone and that young guy, the suicide case they brought in, he'll still be there, he'll live." The door would open and in we'd trail, see who was there, not there and over there, my heroic Dad, barely visible for a mass of tubes and space-age machines, but still there, hanging on, dangling in the twilight zone.

We became a family of people caring for people caring for other people. Mum cared for Dad, holding his hand and whispering soothing single words in her scratchy voice. My brother and sister cared for Mum and Dad. Relatives and friends cared for my brother and sister and Mum. Mum cared for my brother and sister and me. I commuted between Berkshire and Edinburgh. I was running on adrenaline, fuelled by caffeine. It's a wonder I didn't fly back to Edinburgh by myself, never mind riding on an airplane. I suffered sporadic panic attacks, where I was convinced that *I* was going to die. Weight fell off me once again as I regained the look of Twiggy (lucky it was a jockey I was playing.) The sound of my own heart thumping kept me awake at night. The make-up people worked miracles to disguise the dark rings, the angry acne. I was jittery, harum-scarum, almost gave them a nervous breakdown. Still they gently restored me as I crumbled, patched me up when my world was ripped apart.

Two months after my father died the BBC gave us ten days holiday. I thought about going home, felt I ought to go home but I didn't. I had an overwhelming desire to take off on my own, unhindered by anything or anyone. I had been having a recurring image. A dream of sorts? I was naked, always naked, kneeling at the foot of some kind of holy man, some kind of healer dressed in a long robe. He had his hands on my head, I had my face bowed to the ground. I lay crumpled at his feet and he was trying to heal me, to put me together again. Like Humpty-Dumpty, my insides lay shattered on the ground. In the image I was always outside, high up somewhere, warm sun on bare skin. Everything superfluous had been stripped away in this pure place, a sanctuary from the silliness of society. It was a place of safety, a place where nothing need be said.

For my holiday, I headed first to the suffocating heat of Athens to visit a dear friend. Then, alone, I caught a boat to a tiny island called Aegina. At the harbour, I got into a cab. "Where do you want to go?" the driver asked. "Dunno. Please drive anywhere you like until I shout stop." He looked at me as if I was mad. He drove. I had never been to Aegina before. We twisted and slithered alongside a turquoise sea. He kept eyeing me nervously in his mirror. I smiled hoping it would look reassuring and not look like the too-forced smile of a nut. At Marathona Bay I saw a turreted house way high up on the cliff with a sign 'Rooms to Rent'. "Stop!" I yelled.

The room was only £10 a night and had a private balcony with a stunning view over the ocean and beyond. Accessible only by a steep climb up a rocky footpath from the village below, I discovered that nobody else was renting a room there. The English lady who owned the building lived elsewhere. I paid a week's rent and was left alone. (Now, I would think, no way, I'm not staying there on my own, but then, it was perfect. It was paradise.)

Each morning, I stripped naked and sat cross-legged in the sun, wondering what on earth I should be doing to heal the broken-ness inside. Sometimes I would make sounds like "Ommm," sometimes I would dance, wave my arms around like a windmill and hop about wildly, sometimes I would just sit quietly and face the sun and breathe in out deep, deeper!

I thought I was safe from prying eyes because I was so far up the hill. Little did I know that there was a house built even further up the hill, hidden behind a row of cypress, whose balcony overlooked mine. I learned this embarrassing fact when I went to dinner, as I did each night in the little taverna in the village, run by three rather good-looking brothers. One evening they laughed and said "Oh here comes the mad woman. Our neighbour tells us you dance about naked in the sun."

"Yes," I said. "My father has just died."

Memory – Twenty-six years old

I am on a plane returning from Portugal. My Mum is seated in front of me.

We will shortly be arriving in Edinburgh after spending three weeks on the Algarve, a place my parents had been planning to visit before Dad fell ill. It is the first time my mother has been abroad. When we left, on 6 October, directly after my filming ended, she was as excited as a child.

I stare out into a black sky. I am utterly exhausted, have been short-tempered, snappy, with Mum, with everyone. Since my father died, since before that, I have kept going and done what needs to be done. I have learned my lines back to front, I have played my part. Months of filming with 6 a.m. starts, bitter-sweet, moving between worlds of death and life, intensive care, newspaper interviews, make-up consultations and meetings with consultants, funerals, photo-shoots, a big smile like I have not a care in the world (liar!). There is a well of grief bubbling, grief that has been pushed down, ignored whilst I have done what needs to be done. I plan what I will do once we touchdown in Edinburgh. I will go off to the Highlands and rent a remote cottage and have at least a month of peace and quiet. I will see no-one, I will laze in bed and read, I will go for walks, I will not worry about anything anymore, I will …

Suddenly Mum's head slumps forward. She is sick and appears to lose consciousness. I leap up and yell the immortal line – "Is there a doctor on board?" A man comes rushing down the aisle. There is turbulence and the air hostess tells me to sit down. I refuse. The doctor calls for an oxygen tank and quietly tells me that he thinks Mum is having another stroke. "The good news," he says, "is even if she were in hospital, there's little they could do."

I hold her head to my belly and caress her hair. I say it's okay, it's okay, but I am terrified. I think, this is it, this is really it … The plane bumps toward Edinburgh. Everyone is staring. A woman seated nearby asks: "Aren't you the girl from *Trainer*?"

As the plane returns to earth, so does Mum. She opens her eyes and asks in guttural tones: "Vot Happened?" I cannot quite believe this resurrection. My brother and sister are waiting as I wheel Mum in, much to her annoyance, in an airport wheelchair. She has always refused to go anywhere in a wheelchair, but needs must. We want to take her straight to hospital but she protests. We take her home. The next day, under duress, she is admitted to hospital. She remains in the high-dependency neurological unit for the next month. Visions of my Highland cottage have vanished in the mist.

Memory – Twenty-seven years old

Mum is newly out of hospital after the plane episode. The diagnosis is vague, the doctors believe yes, she may have had another stroke or 'something'. Whatever it is, she requires twenty-four hour care.

We curl up on the bed, drink tea, watch telly, chat about Dad. I worry that she cannot express her grief like people who can speak can express their grief. Whenever I mention him her face lights up and she says in her gritty voice: "Best friend, best-est friend," then she laughs, hoots, howls. I say that's it, have a good cry, cry it's okay, 'Hang loose.'

'Hang loose' is a saying we madeup, we use a lot, it sort of means just let it out, let it go, hang loose.

But now I am hanging loose like a zombie, becoming unhinged.

I am desperate to get away for a rest, recover some energy. I suggest I contact a private care agency. Mum hits the roof. She doesn't want a stranger in her house. I don't go. One morning, in the bathroom, I find myself lying on the floor, screaming. It sounds as if the screams are coming from elsewhere. I then calmly get up and telephone my brother who is at work. I tell him in my most dramatic voice: "I think I've just had a nervous breakdown." He says "Oh yes?" I say: "I'm phoning to let you know that I am going away for a few days and I'm arranging some private care for Mum." He says: "Okay. Have a good time." I pack a case. I tell Mum that a nurse is coming for three days, I am going away for a rest. I feel awful guilt doing this, yet still I do it. When the smiley nurse turns up she tells us her name is … Audrey! The irony of the moment is an ice-breaker. When I leave, Audrey (my Mum) is making Audrey (the nurse) a cup of tea. I catch a train to the Yorkshire Wolds. My dear friend Phil collects me from the station, his wife Jen feeds me wholesome meals, I am tucked up in a warm bed and left for hours to sleep. Mugs of tea, toast and compassion greet me when I wake. I thank God for friends such as these. I return to Scotland a new being; nurtured and cared for.

Memory – Twenty-seven years old

Mum tells us that she does not want to be hospitalized if anything else happens to her. "Why Mum, why?" we bleat. "They can help you." She smiles a sad, wry smile, indicates her body and says, "Done."

I ask her if she means that, really means that, that she doesn't want to go to hospital even if she is having some awful attack or something. She nods, then shakes her head of thick silver hair, china blue eyes shining and repeats in her growly voice: "Done." Casually as I can muster, I chirp: "So you're not afraid to die, Mum?" She shrugs comically. "Dead n' gawn. Dead n' gaw – n." Silence. My brother, who has a wonderful dry wit, breaks the moment. From his pocket he takes out a measuring tape and begins to mock measuring up my Mum. We all, including Mum, laugh, but I am worried. Will I really be able to respect my mother's wishes when the moment comes?

The testing moment comes sooner rather than later. Just after New Year, after breakfast, Mum is in bed, pure white, writhing in agony, one clammy hand clutching her chest, groaning.

"I'll call an ambulance."

"No!" she gasps.

"Well, I'm calling the doctor …"

My hand shakes as I dial the number. As I gush the sentence it sounds like a bad joke – "Doctor, doctor, I think my Mum is having a heart-attack, what should I do?" Minutes later, a paramedic van is at our door. I think, oh no, my Mum will kill me. Seconds later, the doctor arrives. (He had called the paramedics.) Mum is refusing to go anywhere, between cries of pain there are audible gasps of "No 'ospital. No 'ospital." We cram around Mum's bed like aliens tentatively examining a new species. I explain that my Mum has previously informed us, her children, if anything happens she doesn't want to go to the hospital. The paramedics say if she doesn't go, she is going to die right here, right now. My stomach heaves. I'm not so brave now. The doctor says, "Please, Mrs Jenkinson, please allow us to take you to the hospital." I plead, "Please Mum, please, please go, they can help you, please, just this time." She doesn't agree or disagree, but raises her eyes impressively to the heavens. Whether this is the heart-attack or simply self-expression noone seems to know but she is drifting and the doctor makes a decision. My Mum is loaded onto a chair and carted off down the path. My aunt, in tears, rushes from the living-room and says, "Audrey, don't let them take her. Don't let them." I pace back and forth, not sure what to do, not sure what I *should* do, please God help me. I am piggy in the middle of the hall, caught between right and wrong, good and bad, hope and despair, unable to tell which is which.

Mum was in hospital for almost a month. It was touch and go. They saved her, but a bit of her heart died.

January in Scotland is chilling and harsh. Dark days and long unrelenting nights.

Mum hated hospital. Her body ached. She was bored. She longed to be home in her own bed.

Not the easiest of patients, the nurses loved Mum because she was such a character. Despite the strokes, she was as sharp as a pin and possessed a wicked sense of humour.

We would pitch up outside visiting hours to check all was okay. I was worried that Mum would be in pain or trying to communicate something to the nurses and they would be unable to understand her. The nurses would greet me with a smile: "Oh, I hear you're an actress, you work in London, your brother has his own business, your sister has three children, your father died last year, your Mum's been telling us."

I would sneak a smile. It was no mean feat for someone who could only utter a limited number of single words to be perfectly understood by strangers. I knew the concerted effort it must have taken on Mum's behalf. What feisty determination to communicate, what an indomitable spirit. She had reclaimed the power of being her own voice in the world and I was immensely proud.

During this time, I took a room in a shared flat close to the hospital. I thought it would allow me a certain freedom. When Mum got out of hospital I could go home each day to help out and then return to my room in the evenings where I hoped I might have some semblance of a 'normal' twenty-something life. A social life would be nice. Perhaps, even, a boyfriend? It had been over three years since I had

had a boyfriend. I missed sex. I missed intimacy (not that the two necessarily go together), but you know the kind of thing, the warmth of flesh against flesh, legs entwined around the legs of another, my back being tickled at midnight. I missed chilling out with friends talking about nothing in particular. I missed fun. I didn't know how to have fun anymore. When I looked in the mirror I saw a face that was so tired, worn out, strained looking, that I began to hate it. I hated my face. No amount of make-up made it brighter. It was dull, ugly. Gaunt cheeks accentuated my nose. I detested my nose. Certain angles that I saw myself at on television made me want to hide. A friend said he thought all I needed was "rest, sea and sun". I thought I needed plastic surgery. I trekked to and from the hospital each day to visit Mum, passing ward upon ward filled with the sick, the dying, and plastic surgery seemed my only hope.

I visited Mum bearing tapes of whale music. It had seemed a good idea at the time, but the whines of the blue whale sounded uncannily like the bleeps of the heart machines. The heart systems soon sounded as if they were going AWOL. I took in talking books. I took in Andrew Lloyd Webber, for God's sake! Mum was not impressed. She hated the hospital and nothing could make it better. One day when I visited, her face lit up and she announced: "Ome." Surprised, I asked, They're letting you go home? She pursed her lips, grinned "Aye." Later that day, she discharged herself.

By the end of February she was back. My brother had taken her out for a delicious lunch to a posh hotel and next thing she was sprawled unconscious across the table. The hotel immediately called an ambulance. (Mind, I don't really see how my brother could have said, excuse me, please don't bother.) We, her three children, assembled at the infirmary and waited anxiously for news. There was nothing we could do but sit and stare into the awful lukewarm polystyrene coffee. Finally a doctor emerged who looked barely out of his teens. I wanted to shout, "fetch an adult, fetch an adult, this is my Mum we're talking about …" He told us Mum had been successfully resuscitated but that it was a major heart attack and she wasn't out of the woods yet. She was on her way to the coronary intensive care unit. Mum had survived, but another chunk of her heart had died. We thanked him and made our way through a maze of grey corridors, searching for signs.

The next two months were a roller-coaster ride. Mum, in hospital, had bad days and good. One minute we were prepared for the worst, the next minute she would astound us by bouncing back. Life was full of twists and turns and blind bends. Anxiety to relief, surrender to hope, letting go and gripping tighter as the next wave came crashing down before I had time to draw breath from the first.

I was shortly due to return to London to begin shooting a second series of *Trainer*. They had axed half the original cast and re-vamped the new series to be 'sexier and steamier'. My Mum was in intensive care. Déjà-vu. Father forgive me.

From a payphone in the infirmary, I called the producer. I don't know how coherent I was. I think I told him my mother was dying, and that I didn't see how I could leave. "I understand," he replied. "But scripts are written, your parts been built up, we need you." Did I want to act in a television show? Yes. Did I want to leave my Mum? No. A schizophrenic moment was resolved by compromise. If they cut down my part in the first three episodes the BBC could delay my scheduled start date for filming. I agreed.

After two and a bit months, Mum got out of hospital. As she left the nurses hugged and kissed her, several in tears. They had grown very fond of her, in awe of her boomerang spirit. She shook each of their hands with her good left hand and thanked them. We left gifts and took Mum home.

My brother was living at home but the demands of keeping his business afloat meant early starts and long hours. I was due to film a television series at the other end of the country. My sister had her hands full coping with three growing children. What on earth to do? Refuge came in the form of an aunt. By chance she was looking for a part-time job and my brother seized the opportunity. He organized for her to come in during the days to help in the home and be with Mum. This arrangement worked well. There was none of the 'no stranger in my house' argument. I headed to Berkshire with a new lightness in my being, if not my backside.

I realised with horror that many months had passed since I last squeezed into my jockey pants. After the first series had ended, I had been full of great ideas about how I would go to the gym, take care of myself, be blooming lovely and radiant for the next series. In reality, I had been so psychologically and physically exhausted that, at every opportunity, I had collapsed in front of the fire stuffing myself with tea and chocolate biscuits. I looked about as radiant as an Eskimo.

That summer settled into a routine of filming and phoning home. I would phone home sometimes three, four times a day. The family I was staying with nicknamed me E.T. – 'phone home, Aud-ree'. To my joy, Mum's health, for the most part, stabilized. On the phone she would tell me about her day. On good days, she'd be taken out for lunch; by cousins, brother, sister, aunts, uncles, friends, sometimes even my friends. There'd be runs in the car or delight! a trip to the shops. (Since the stroke, Mum had developed a love of trying and buying though it took ages to get the darn outfit on and off. Mum was in her element, her dressers on their knees.) Other days, if nothing much had happened I would get a resounding one-word answer to my question: "How're you today, Mum?" "Bo-rrrrd." Since the stroke, she hated staying in.

After a hectic day filming, with dusk falling, I would gather up the cheeky Jack Russell terriers I lodged with and make my way up onto the Downs. I would walk for miles disturbed by nothing but nature. How I loved it up here, walking in the hazy twilight.

Across my path baby bunnies dashed to and fro, the dogs scurrying comically after them with (thankfully) no joy. The light caught between day and night, glowed magical, bathing the earthly world in the ethereal. I would walk, on and on, sinking into the stillness. Broken only by bird-song, this stillness seemed to wrap itself around me, protect me as I walked. On and on over the Downs, not wanting to break the spell, I would walk. The sight of a mare grazing with her foal, a kitten snuggled in the grass, the simple beauty of the evening would move me and I would often find my eyes wet with silent tears. On I would walk, trying to imagine my life, a future, without my Mum; it was unimaginable.

During this summer I met a boy I liked. I hadn't had a boyfriend for four years and it was exciting to have met someone I finally, as they say in Scotland, *fancied*. He was American. He was self-assured and super-confident and a lotta fun. I was fragile, defensive, and seriously not-a-lotta fun. His job involved travelling to Europe. What with my filming and days off going back to Scotland, it was amazing that we managed to co-ordinate a couple of dinner dates. Thereafter our 'relationship' became of the telephone kind. As I flew from Heathrow to see Mum he would be sailing in from Spain. When I was filming he would be seventy miles away working. When I had an afternoon off, he would have a morning off. Talk about frustrating!

44

We casually discussed the possibility of going to France together at the end of our respective contracts. We would have two weeks in October before his return to America.

One day, at the end of September, I called home. Mum sounded excited.

"Coooze," she gushed.

"Coos?" I asked, puzzled, thinking cows, milk, countryside?

"Crrroose."

"Cruise?"

"Aye."

"Who's going on a cruise? I asked, thinking, must be one of our neighbours.

"Yoo."

"Me ?"

"ME."

"You?"

"Yoo n'me!" She bellowed down the phone, delighted.

Memories – October 1992

Mum and I are sipping tea on a cliff terrace in Sorrento, the Bay of Naples shimmering in the distance. It is a terrace I once saw in a magazine when I was a teenager. It looked like one of those places that you had to be 'somebody' before you went there. Like they might have a sign outside that said No Entry Unless … I dreamed of going there one day, some day, but probably never would have. Mum is basking in the warm sun. She looks like a movie star in her tinted sunglasses and white wide-brimmed sun hat. Waiters in white run around with pots of tea and mouth-watering pastries. This is the life, I tell Mum. She nods and repeats in her growly tones: "This – is – life." She has missed 'the' out. She always does. The wee-est word, the hardest to say. "The" I say, and she rolls her eyes and lights up.

Mum and I are winding our way down the narrow cobbled lanes of southern Italian hill villages, we are shouting "Ciao!" and waving to curious schoolchildren. We are eating fresh delicious pasta in outdoor cafés where Italians wave their hands in the air as they ask, "Mama?" I nod. "Ah, bellisima." In the streets, in the cafés, in the houses with open doors, there is evidence of the importance of family, of generations caring for one another. When we set off down the steep slopes I struggle to hang onto Mum's wheelchair, we are in danger of 'vertical speedygonzales'. Within seconds two strong Italian men are by my side, taking over, steering 'Mama' wherever she wants to go. Mama is Queen Bee as her escorts flit her from one curio shop to the next.

Mum and I are sailing along the Amalfi coastline on a catamaran, the luxury villas of the rich and famous scattered along the coast. Mum raises her face to the sun, enjoying the warm breeze on her skin, the wind in her hair, oh, what freedom! She has never been sailing before. Her wheelchair bobs sharply to the rhythm of the waves, up, down, up, down, I hang on to the handles ever tighter for fear of Mum going for a quick dip.

She is in a wheelchair – only – for the purpose of this trip. On the big ship *Canberra*, it has been agreed pride should be cast aside in favour of actually getting around. Trying to walk on a lolling ship is difficult enough.

We had been looking forward to the sailing trip but it almost didn't happen. The only way aboard the catamaran was across an extremely narrow free-floating wooden gangplank with only two thin strips of rope to cling to either side. The tiny gangplank was bouncing like a trampoline, such was the choppiness of the sea. There was no way Mum, who could barely walk unaided, could negotiate her way across. We were disappointed. We were about to leave when suddenly an actor in the *Canberra's* theatre troupe noticed us. Projecting his voice to the hilt he announced he needed volunteers to get Mum on board. Within seconds, people started filing back off the catamaran onto the quayside, roughly around fifteen folk, mostly men. Another group was assembling on board. I was told to stand aside. The group on the quayside crouched down, like a rugby scrum, and gripped wheels, handles, anything. On the count of three Mum's wheelchair with Mum perched atop was suddenly airborne. I watched in awe and horror as Mum tilted back and forth at precarious angles. The men heaved and struggled and puffed (Mum was a solid woman) as, with considerable effort, they hoisted her ever higher. I saw knees buckle and lips being bit as, with an almighty strength they passed Mum in her chair out over the edge of the sea. Dozens of hands reached skyward to catch Mum on the other side. The catamaran, rising and falling with the swell was a tricky landing spot but the sea of hands held tight, stretched to their limit, clinging tightly to their cargo. I watched thinking God, what if they drop her? What if she rolls out? She'll go straight down belly-buster style into the water. But Mum, suspended on her mid-air throne, was apparently unafraid. I could hear her repeating "Right! Right! Right!" in encouragement as she was slowly manoeuvred down, down, down. A huge cheer erupted as four wheels made contact with the floor of the catamaran complete with one chuffed Mum still sitting comfortably. I burst into tears, not only with relief but because it was, and will remain, one of the most moving sights of my life.

When Mum had suggested a cruise it had seemed a crazy idea. I can't drive. Mum wasn't allowed to fly. The cruises departed from the other end of the country. The train journey would be almost a day, Edinburgh to Kings Cross, across London to Waterloo, and on to Southampton. What about trying to walk on a high-speed train? Even perfectly balanced people end up in someone's lap. Ever tried peeing on a train? Oops! What would happen if Mum took ill en route? How would we get across London when Mum couldn't get her right leg high enough to climb into the back of a black cab? How could we transport our luggage when I needed to link my arm through Mum's when we walked? The list was long. If we had done the logical 'sensible' thing, we'd never have gone. But who wants to be sensible when it's a matter of life and death?

We had sought the opinion of the family doctor. I had asked him, should we stay, should we go? He replied: "Well, exertion of any kind can put a strain on the heart." My heart sank. "But," he added, "it could as easily happen if your Mum stayed within these four walls and did nothing." The 'it' being … what? … a stroke, heart attack, death?

So it seemed our choice was – stay within these four walls, take it easy and wait for death to visit, he's on his way, maybe not today or tomorrow but he is overdue. Or go, see, do a little, dream a little, have an adventure, a trip of a lifetime. Death may come quicker but when he does you can say look, look where I have been, what I have seen …

I thought, I am twenty-seven, there will be other chances for me to go off to France with handsome American men, there may never be another chance for me to go cruising with my Mum. Today, tomorrow, she may not be well enough or dead.

My brother dropped us at Waverley Station and we were off. Like Thelma and Louise, there was abandon in our souls as we sailed across the Bay of Biscay. Mum was a smoker. Let her smoke. She loved good food. Let her eat to her heart's content. She wanted to go on a cruise. Yes let's do it. Let us indulge, do anything and everything, let us *live*. Let's stay up and count the stars, let's sip whisky and champagne, let's dance at the disco 'til 3am, whirling your chair this way and that, yes, let's push the boat out, plunge in head-first. So what if this trip of a lifetime costs a lifetime's savings? You can't take it with you.

The moment I surrendered my fear I felt the chains slip away. In accepting that whatever happened happened my worried heart breathed free. I trusted life, death. We knew the rules of the game, knew the risks, the consequences. We knew that Mum may not survive the trip but she would have a great time dying. If she was about to pop off any second in dreich Auld Reekie, why not upgrade to the romantic island of Elba or the star-spangled streets of Monaco or within the ancient walls of a castle in Palma?

As the *Canberra* sailed out of the Bay of Naples, Mum and I stood arm in arm on the deck gazing at the array of twinkling lights illuminated in a black sky. "Die!" Mum suddenly said. I asked her, "What?" You want to die? She shook her head, cocked her head towards the lights and repeated "Die".

I said: "You think you're going to die? Are you in pain, are you sore?" She made a face as if to say dumbo and growled louder like a grumpy bear: "Die – nipples – die." Now I'm completely lost. A woman standing next to us turned and in a hushed tone said, "Excuse me, I don't mean to interrupt, but perhaps your Mum is saying once you've seen the Bay of Naples you can die? It's a famous saying …" Mum nodded and gave the woman the thumbs-up sign. I said indignantly: "Well, I've never heard of that. Who said that?" Mum screwed her bright eyes up in concentration, then shrugged och never mind and we stood in silence, arms around each other, until the Bay of Naples was engulfed in darkness.

On the second last day of the cruise, at eleven o'clock at night, Mum suffered a heart-attack. They rushed her down to the ship's hospital where a stern doctor in a paisley dressing-gown attached her to bits and pieces and injected her with syringes full of God knows what. I stepped out onto the deck and prayed. Please, please God, take her now, don't let her suffer any more, I can handle it tonight, please, if you take her tonight, I can handle it.

Next morning a sprightly Mum was sitting in an armchair. She had survived but a lot more of her heart had died.

The doctor told her she should stay in the ship's hospital until we docked at Southhampton but she would hear none of it. She had a luxury cabin one floor up and that's where she was going. The ship's hospital was lifeless and stank of disinfectant. She had paid a lot of money for a little comfort and she had one day left to enjoy it. The doctor indignantly told her that if she moved that one floor up to her luxury cabin she was seriously endangering her health. Up to me, Mum nodded. "Me – my – life." Trying to scare her, he snapped, "You could die". "No prob-lum," shrugged Mum. "Dead and gone." And with that she got up, hobbled to the door and was off …

When we docked at Southampton my brother was waiting. He had driven through the night. We settled back for the long journey to Edinburgh but Mum was keen to sightsee. We turned off near where I had been filming *Trainer* and had an ad-hoc tour of the area. This is the yard where we filmed, this is the cottage where I stayed,

this is the dung-heap I got thrown into in my first episode, remember?
We drove to the village pub in East Ilsley, the one used for the filming,
where Mum had seen me on celluloid tearfully shuffle food around
my plate, being teased as overweight by a bunch of unmerciful lads.
Mum, as if in defence of her wee lass, surveys a cast photo grinning
from the walls and loudly declares me skinny, too skinny as I laugh
shhh, and tuck in.

Memory – Twenty-eight years old

"No 'ospital."

"Please Mum …"

"No 'ospital."

"I think you …"

"Tired. So, so tired."

"But …"

"Done. Finished."

"Listen …"

"No 'ospital. No doctor. Promise." Silence.

"I promise."

"Thank-oo. Cup of tea?"

I stick the kettle on as Mum sings along to the theme tune of *Neighbours*.

The phone rang. It was Steve, owner of the cottage where I had lodged whilst filming. "Someone called here. Wanted to know if you were interested in doing a National Theatre tour. Called a while back. Sorry. I forgot."

It was my own fault. I should have got an agent … should have … it was probably cast by now … I called anyway.

"Audrey, yes, we were trying to get hold of you. Sorry, we've now cast Kate Beckinsdale …"

I hung up. Disappointed. Then relief. I didn't have to choose. Funny how things work out.

The next time Mum has a heart-attack my sister and I hide in the front room because we cannot bear to see the agony, the pain. Still nothing can smother the cries, the moans. They go on and on. This is killing me. This is ridiculous. Why don't we just call the doctor? I have made a promise.

Over weeks, weeks, what was left of her heart got weaker, weaker, and now other organs began to fail. It was unfair. Why couldn't my Mum just have a massive attack, just one big hit, instead of this torturous drawn-out affair? C'mon God, play the game. Quit pussy-footing around, just do it. Just take her.

There was daily sickness, basins of sickness.

One lunch-time, as I was carrying such a basin to dispose of in the bathroom the phone rang.

"Hello?"

"Hey Aud."

The boy from America was in Australia. He had asked me to come over, I had told him I couldn't. He had sounded annoyed, said, "What about your life? What about you?" I thought, it's easy to say what about you when you're not me.

"How're you doin'?"

"Fine. Mum's really ill. It's bad. She's just been sick."

"Sorry to hear that."

Pause.

"What're you wearing?"

"Eh?"

"Bet you look cute."

It took me a moment to clock that he was on the other side of the world, quite drunk and … hmm … it was that time of night. I hung up.

I flushed the sickness away, some place far away and how I longed to disappear too, sucked down to the other side of the world. I would hide in the arms of a shallow man, sink into his wetness, bathe my boiling skin in a cool clear ocean. I would scream to the brooding storm "Come, come, you can't scare me". I would turn back the tide rising in my mother's chest. I would drown the giant rats seeping out of bedroom walls. I would send on the breeze a breath of fresh air.

Air for the breathless.

In the suffocating depths.

Air.

An animal wouldn't be kept alive like this. It wouldn't be allowed. The person would be fined. Jailed.

We were there in the room, wrapped our arms around her and whispered,

"Go … go to Dad

… go now …

it's time."

She died, as was her wish, in her own bed.

We played *My Way* at her funeral. She would have liked that.

I wake on 23 January 1993. It takes a moment before the shock hits. My father is dead. My mother is dead.

I am past caring.

Part 2

PAST CARING

Past Caring

"Life has to be lived forward, but understood backward."
George Bernard Shaw

As humans, it is necessary for us to give interpretations and explanations to events, in order to make life bearable. This is not to say this is a bad thing. This is a good thing, otherwise life would be unbearable.

As humans, we are constantly evolving. How we feel today may not be the same as tomorrow, or next week, or next year. We may have new insights, shift our view, our understanding of ourselves, of others. We connect feelings of then and now. Our stories grow, develop and become something else.

The following stories are snapshots in time. They are how the person felt that day. They are reflective of an individual's understanding of their life in that moment. Present and past tense are often interwoven, as we struggle to make sense of past loss and new beginnings. Through sharing our stories we come to understand ourselves, and help others to understand themselves too.

Although the stories are relevant to past carers, they touch on basic human emotion and will therefore speak to people going through a major life change such as divorce or redundancy or those whose loved ones have died suddenly.

Most of the interviews involve one person talking. Some are a conglomerate of voices that speak about a similar theme. I have also included my own memories of past caring. Some stories tell of how caring for the dying teaches us about ourselves: the new values we take into our lives, the way we look at the world differently.

Sometimes I did an interview and went back several years later to see how the person was doing. How was life progressing – or not? Some sections are simply questions and answers. I had fun asking the question and letting the answers speak for themselves.

Let's just start with the word **carer**. It sounds a completely dull, unsexy word.

I asked a group of healthy people (who had never been involved in caring for an ill person) what is the first image or word that springs to mind when I say the word **carer**:
- A white uniform
- My boyfriend, Fraser
- A person who empties bedpans
- A wee wifey
- Rubber gloves and disinfectant
- Someone old
- My Mum
- Is this a joke?
- D'you mean *career*?
- Wheelchairs
- I care for you but I'm not your carer – am I?
- Blue-rinse biddies
- Someone who devotes their time to another
- A martyr
- Social worker
- Jesus sandals and long woolly sweaters

Carer – noun (according to the dictionary)
a family member or paid helper who regularly looks after a sick, elderly or disabled person.
Care – noun
serious attention and thought; caution to avoid damage or loss, protection, supervision, worry, anxiety.
Care – verb
Feel concern, interest, affection or liking, take charge of; see to the safety or well-being of; deal with.

Just for fun I looked up:
Career – noun
An occupation undertaken for a significant period of a person's life, usually with progress; (before another noun) working with long-term commitment in a particular profession.

I'm worried about carers and what people think about carers. The following letter is from Gordon:

Dear Audrey,

I have just read the National Carers Magazine and your intentions to write a book on past caring. You may be of the opinion that a great deal has already been written on the subject of 'Caring' and this is true within certain restraints but the complete story has never been uncovered so yet again the true picture is torn in half.

In discussing caring, we have a tendency to omit what could be considered, quite wrongly, as being offensive, embarrassing, sickening, shocking, painful or unpleasant. If we photograph the invalid and the carer together then more often than not the resulting picture is a big broad smile that gives the viewer a very misleading impression of caring.

Of course the invalid would be too embarrassed to talk about or be pictured in a number of situations but in this instance we are discussing the carer's problems and not the invalid's problems. I have a vast amount of sympathy and understanding for the invalid's feelings and their point of view but that does not mean that the carer's problems should be hidden, out of sight and never recorded.

As an example, picture the carer cleaning excrement off the front room carpet or off the stairs or standing behind the invalid with a bucket. Picture the carer washing excrement off the patient's body or from their clothes. What about the lifting and carrying, the complete loss of freedom and leisure time, the financial loss to the carer, the continuous non-stop talking about the invalid's condition and extremely important to me, the mind-destroying sexual frustration. We have now reduced the carer to little more than a mechanical robot.

If you were a hospital patient laying alongside another patient who was continuously moaning and groaning and despite your sympathy and possibly after shedding a few tears for the patient how long would it be before you requested a move? Would it be after just a few hours, a few days, a few months or many years?

Yes, we have all lost part of our lives. These strains and pressures I have described as a carer now encompass my entire life. I am sixty-one years of age and my wife has suffered the complaint of Multiple Sclerosis for the past eighteen years. She is severely disabled.

I married at the age of thirty. There followed the birth of two wonderful boys, we had a nice home, holidays at the seaside, Christmas presents, birthday presents. I was employed as a Production and Stock Control Supervisor within a medium sized engineering company. I enjoyed my work and regarded it as a pleasing pastime rather than compulsory slavery.

Yes, I do feel deeply hurt and very angry at having been cheated out of my normal life. I feel angry at the loss of work and the loss of salary over the last eighteen years. I am virtually a prisoner in my own home due to my wife's illness. My life dominated and controlled by my wife's medical complaint, twenty-four hours a day, seven days a week, year after year, without change and no future. At the same time I do have a great amount of sympathy for my wife and when she falls or hurts herself it also hurts me and as I place my arms around her to comfort her, the tears often roll down my face.

As I previously mentioned, like any adult individual I yearn for a partner who enjoys the same sexual desires. I sometimes do try to involve my wife in one way or the other in some form of intimacy but with little success.

I am sorry to go on about the sexual frustration but it is often a part of a carer's life that the mainstream organisations tend to avoid talking about or choose to deliberately overlook. If the sexual act is discussed at all it is discussed in a very clinical way to make it sound more like instructions on how to repair a motor car than sexual intercourse. Thing is, who can we talk to and where do we draw the line?

For people past caring, it's like losing their job. A job they may have been doing for most of their life. Although it is not recognised or respected as such in our society, past carers have lost what has become, indirectly, their career. For many years they have been working with long-term commitment as a care-giver.

An issue that came up time and time again was 'the gap' - 'the hole' - this incredible void that exists after the caring stops. Overnight, with no warning and no time to prepare, the job ends. Redundancy notice is served. And there isn't even a gold clock or an attractive financial package to ease the fact that your services are no longer required.

Freedom comes with grief. Bitter-sweet. Death gives way to re-birth.

The most terrifying day for many prisoners is the day they get their freedom back. If they have been locked up for years, the prison has become their familiar territory, their safety. When something is unfamiliar, it feels frightening. So too can long-term caring create a loop of dependency. At first you may resent your life as a carer. Then you get used to it. It becomes familiar, all-consuming. And finally you depend on it. The writer, George Eliot, had a difficult time caring for her father. But after his death and a longed for holiday she wrote: "My return to England is anything but joyous to me, for old associations are rather painful than otherwise to me. We are apt to complain of the weight of duty, but when it is taken from us, and we are left at liberty to choose, we find that the old life was easier."

Some people may know no other life than caring. Ursula, a remarkable young woman, cared for her mother Margaret from the tender age of ten. Now thirty-two years of age and five years past caring, Ursula talks about how her mother's wish for freedom brought her face-to-face with her own fear of freedom. Ursula's father left home when she was a child. She cared from age ten through those teenage years and early twenties, when life is, ought to be, an adventure in breaking free, experimenting, spreading wings. It's an age of studying, college, jobs abroad, dream careers. It's an age of discovering ourselves and others, forging friendships, relationships, discovering sex, lust, love. It's an age of heartbreak and headiness, where we hope our parents guide us but are not involved, give us space to develop in the world but keep a caring eye out for us, healthy neglect.

Ursula was twenty when she married John, thirty-nine. They have a son, Scott, eight. I interviewed Ursula twice for this book, once a year past caring and again at five years past caring.

* * *

Ursula's Story - one year past caring

I left school age ten. It was legal – Mum arranged it through a scheme called Education Otherwise. I was dyslexic. It was agreed it would be more beneficial for Mum to teach me at home. Mum was very intelligent, well educated. Things went well at first, although I did miss going to school, and seeing friends. But as Mum's condition (Parkinson's) deteriorated she became very depressed. I was doing more and more to help her. In those six years, aged ten to sixteen, I had three visits from social services to see how things were going but nobody came from the Local Authority to see how I was getting on with my education.

I was sixteen when it really sunk in that I would be caring as an adult for Mum. One of my friends said "don't do it Ursula". But if I didn't, then who would? They say everyone has a choice but it didn't look that way at the time. It seemed a natural progression but not one that I was looking forward to. I was dreading it. I got very depressed at the thought of what might lie ahead. The future looked bleak.

As a teenager I had such a low opinion of myself. I let boys use me for sex. I thought, that way they'll like me, they'll call me again, because what else can I offer them? I'm a carer. I am boring, boring, boring. I have no idea who Wham are, I've never heard of Duran Duran, I wear my Mum's old clothes. They're not going to be interested in me. Of course, they never did call me again, and this seemed to confirm my belief that I was boring and uninteresting.

On a rare occasion, if I could get someone to sit with Mum, I would go to a local disco. I enjoyed a night out, but there was always part of me worrying; is Mum okay? Will the sitter cope? I couldn't go out regularly like my friends. I soon dropped out of being 'one of the crowd'. It made me sad. Lonely.

Age seventeen, I fancied a career in catering or hotel management. I enrolled on several courses. I enjoyed college and meeting people. But it was hard to go in every day if Mum was unwell. Or I'd arrive at college only to be told the day centre (where Mum went) had been on the phone: "There's a problem." I had to rush away. In the end it got so difficult, I abandoned the idea of following any kind of training at that time.

I met my husband John on one of those courses. I told him, "I come with a package." Normally men were off *tout de suite* when they heard I had to look after Mum. John was different. He accepted me for who I was.

Over the years of caring for Mum, it has been tough for John and Scott too. Some days were very divided, Mum crying for help and aid, Scott crying for his bottle and nappy changing. He was very close to his grandmother and seeing her dying was traumatic for him. Scott and I had a lot of catching up to do in our mother/son relationship because I just didn't have time for him before. We managed to get a place at Winston's Wish, they do a very helpful two-day session for bereaved children and their parents. It really helped us through the first rough stages, I mean, you always get them, even now …

When Mum passed away my hormones, emotions, everything went haywire. I faced a major identity crisis. I had lost my job, a job I had done all my life. I didn't know who I was anymore. Since ten years of age I had been a carer. Over the years, my personality had gradually become an extension of my Mum's. Suddenly she was gone and I was stranded. Mixed-up, confused. I needed time, time to myself, to discover who I was, but John was going through a bad period of unemployment and money was tight, red bills piling up. My Carer's allowance had stopped the day after Mum died. I was absolutely knackered, yet I had to find a job ... but doing what?

With no educational qualifications and no experience 'in the workplace' I tried for various jobs, but didn't even get to the interview stage. The first thing employers want to know is: "Have you got this? Have you got that?" We had no food in the cupboard. I was desperate. I finally got a job as a cleaner but automatically came down with one illness after the other – flu, chest infection, colds – it seemed all the illnesses I had repressed over the years when I had to keep going suddenly emerged and knocked my body for six. I felt like I'd been run over by a truck, every muscle ached. I tried to keep going but my body refused. In the end I lost the job due to taking so much time off.

I got another job at a Home Care Agency, but the minute I walked in and saw this old lady wriggling and contorted in a chair, she reminded me so much of Mum, I just couldn't take it. I used to come out of there and cry and cry and cry ...

The social services told me I wasn't eligible for unemployment benefits because I had never worked. It seemed unreal. I had looked after Mum for seventeen years. I and others like me save our Government billions. If I had not cared, I would have been able to work and would never have been in this position to begin with.

I was in their office one day, crying, begging for something, anything. I was totally skint, and they kept saying sorry, there's nothing we can do.

Finally I got up to leave. A lady followed me. She said "I believe your story is genuine, I hope this helps," and handed me a twenty pound note. I was so shocked I didn't think to ask her name. I would love to see her again to thank her properly. To be given twenty pounds by a complete stranger – it restored my faith in human kindness.

My concentration has been shot to pieces since Mum died. I find it difficult to focus on anything. It's as if I'm still waiting for something awful to happen, for Mum to be screaming for help. Life is overturned. I'm all at sea, restless, twitchy, can't settle. It's a horrible feeling, panicky...

Friends keep saying, "Get a job Ursula, you need the money," but my body feels shattered. I think I need time. I was in town the other day and I went into a café and had a coffee and a read of the paper. What a luxury! Never before had I been able to do that.

In this period of re-adjustment I've had feelings I've never experienced in my life, quite frightening feelings of violence. One day I was sitting on the sofa and felt real darkness, despair. Life seemed completely overwhelming. I started screaming and screaming and I couldn't stop. On and on, these blood-curling shrieks came pouring out of me. It was like 'after all these years of caring, look at my life!'

You feel so invisible, feel like nobody recognises what you've done. Not the State. Not potential employers. Not even your own family sometimes. I felt abandoned. Sore. Raw. I had to really struggle to stop myself smashing the house up. I wanted to. I wanted to punch and smash and destroy everything in the room, and I wanted to punch certain individuals too. I imagined me punching them one by one and the images were violent, really violent. It was so unlike me, so unlike Ursula. I was scared of all this violence pouring out of me. In the end I phoned the Samaritans and they came out to see me. They looked at me and said, "Oh my goodness, you are in a bad way, aren't you?"

As a carer it's easier to go along with things, you're so tired, you don't have the energy to argue, someone wants something, you fetch it, someone wants you to do something, you do it. Since Mum died, I stand up for myself more. My relationship with John has changed a bit. John wants me to have another baby. But I don't want to be tied down again. John says he doesn't think it's fair for Scott to be an only child. But I don't think it's fair to push me into doing something that I know will do me in again. I just couldn't cope. I've had enough of sleepless nights, changing nappies, caring for someone round the clock. I suppose if I had never been a carer, this issue would never have arisen.

You know what I would love? I would love to have a career. I have applied to go to college part-time to study for GCSE's. I know it's a rocky road ahead, I know I'll be competing with eighteen year olds, but I am determined to better my education. All my life I've been doing for others. Now it's my turn to do something for me. I was so nervous when I went for the interview for college I was literally shaking. When I got a place I couldn't believe it. I know it sounds funny but I want to go further than people would ever expect of me. A friend said "I never even thought you'd get into college, Ursula." Well I want to prove to folk there's more to me than cleaning and cooking and caring. What's more, I want to prove it to myself.

I have nothing against cleaners, but I don't want to be forty and cleaning up other people's shit. When I was in Woolworths cleaning the toilets, the stench of urine and poo was unbearable. The final straw was when I went to use the toilet brush to clean the loo and saw someone had poohed in there. I thought – NO, no more! I must get an education even if it kills me.

Facing a future where I feel so far behind everybody else is scary. But caring for Mum has taught me that you don't know what's going to happen to you so you must make the most of your life. You may make mistakes, nobody's perfect, but if you don't take a risk, you'll never know. Life is like walking a tightrope, you've got to keep going, even though it's uncertain. A carer may not realise it, but they have tremendous courage. I think of the nights that I used to go into Mum's bedroom and find her in bed with urine and stools all over her body and in her hair. Most people would run a mile. It takes courage to face it, to smell it, to muck in, to deal with it. That same courage is what keeps me going as I try to re-build my life today.

Mum tried to commit suicide on several occasions. Mentally she was all there, but physically she suffered from advanced Parkinson's, she'd had a stroke, a bad hyatus hernia, ulcerated eyes, had difficulty eating, swallowing, she'd wasted away to less than seven stone. She felt life wasn't worth it. She tried to overdose on her medication. Practically paralysed, her hands useless, the tablets never got near her mouth but spilled over the bed. We found her like that. I could understand her wishes but I couldn't stand by and do nothing. I felt guilty, like ... I'm about to let somebody *die*? I know it's selfish wanting to hang onto people and if it were me lying there, I'd want to go too. Laugh is, I know my son Scott wouldn't let me. Look at him nodding there. He'd keep me going, just the way I kept Mum going!

On several occasions, Mum asked me to help end her life.

I could see, logically, it would have made sense, been a good thing if I had been the type of person who was capable of helping her. But emotionally, it was too hard. Perhaps, if the laws were changed, I would like to think I might have had the courage. But I have a young son I want to see grow up. I couldn't be a mother in prison.

Also, there were the what ifs ... what if Mum had turned round and said "thank goodness you didn't finish me off yesterday, today I want to live ...?"

I'm sure Mum thought her being alive was a pain not only for her but for me too. I'm sure her thinking was, if I'm dead Ursula can get on with her life. It was a hellish life in a lot of ways, being a carer, but I still had my Mum. Though the roles were reversed (one year she sent me a Mother's Day Card, saying thanks Ursula for taking care of me), she was my Mum and friend. I'd sit on the bed beside her, we'd chat, joke, I could tell her my worries, get advice. I loved her to bits. Miss her like chronic.

Past caring is a hellish life in a lot of ways too. Caring is like being in a cocoon. It's the pain and pleasure syndrome. Trapped yet protected. The pleasure and pain of being in a cocoon is sometimes better than being out of the cocoon. The screen broken, the world is waiting … and the thought of having to go back into a world you have not been a part of for many years is terrifying.

I now see that I was scared. Very scared. What would happen to me after Mum had gone?

* * *

This is a question carers often ask themselves. But the most dreaded question is asked by others … "So what are you going to do now?"

I asked a selection of past carers, "what's your pet please-don't-say line?"

"Oh, it's a blessing really, that they're gone, you can get on with your own life now." (*er, what life exactly?*)

Myrna shared with me how she filled the void for the first year following her husband's death. She had been caring for her husband Ian, who suffered from heart problems, for seven years. With Ian's death, not only did Myrna have to cope with her grief, but also the loss of purpose in her own life.

Myrna's Story

Heathrow Airport.

I've just said goodbye to my son. He is returning to Canada, where he has made his home, with his wife and two children. This morning we buried my husband, his father. I have said goodbye to my son.

What will I do now?

How am I to get through the rest of the day, the rest of my life? I have no other family in England to support me ... and I cannot lean too heavily on my son. He has his own grief to deal with – not only for his father, but, for himself, as he lives with the recent knowledge he has an incurable brain tumour.

I catch the Airline bus into London. On impulse, I get off at Knightsbridge. I go into Harrods. In a daze, I wander aimlessly from department to department. Anything to delay going home to an empty house. All too soon, a tannoy announcement echoes, muffled – they are closing! It seems as if I have only just arrived. I don't want to leave. I have no choice.

I exit onto the cold street packed with busy commuters, all rushing, frenetic, all going somewhere. But where will I go?

It is raining. I walk and walk. I arrive at my front door. I can't delay it any longer. The emptiness – silence – engulfs me, like a tidal wave. I want to run out again.

I have no idea what to do with myself. My husband is dead. For seven years my life revolved around his life, his needs. My husband was my life. I don't know what to do with this emptiness. In this emptiness I have no purpose. My husband needed me. Now I need him.

I am free ...

Can't think. Can't settle ... don't know what to do ... I am desperate.

That night, I don't sleep a wink. I make endless cups of tea. I rise at dawn. I get washed and dressed and leave the house as quickly as possible.

I go shopping – M&S, Monsoon, Next – crawling through rails

of clothes buying, buying, buying. I make sure I pay by credit card and that all the goods can be returned if 'not suitable'. When it gets dark and the shops are pulling down their shutters, I return home.

The emptiness is still there but now it is easier to bear. I have a purpose. I have lots of new clothes to try on …

The next day I get up early. I catch the bus into town. I have the clothes with me. I will go to a different area to return them. I go to the branches of the chain stores in Bromley. That afternoon I go to Kingston and buy more clothes from the same shops. That evening I go home and try them on. Tomorrow I will get up early and return them … and so I will have a purpose to the day, a reason to get up in the morning … and so I will not have to sit within these four empty walls not knowing what to do or where to turn … and so my life went on … for a year. For a whole year, that was the pattern of my life. That's when I say thank God for the credit card, as all the clothes were charged to VISA and credited the next day. Without the credit card, who knows, maybe I would have stolen the goods.

That first year I didn't give a damn about my appearance. I wore no make-up, let my hair grow, scraped it back in a ponytail. I put on over a stone in weight through comfort eating. Inside I felt dead, I just got through the day on automatic pilot. I washed myself more out of habit than conscious choice. I neglected the house, I had no interest in it. I didn't invite anyone round anyway, as I was always out. I just couldn't bear to be in the house on my own.

CRUSE saved me. I discovered CRUSE and for the first time I realised I was not alone. It was such a relief to find that I could talk to someone who completely understood how I felt.

Friends (from before my husband's death) had not been able to give me a lot of support, simply because they could not identify with my situation at all. They still had their partners, their lives continued same as usual. I was in a state of upheaval. I now found their conversations trivial, superficial. I realised that before my husband's death I must have been a good listener, but now I was the one who needed to talk, it seemed they just couldn't cope with it, especially as it was about a subject that frightened them – death.

Through CRUSE (CRUSE Bereavement Care), who gave me counselling, I have managed to re-build my life. If I am having a bad day, I pick up the phone and ring another member of CRUSE. I know with them I will be able to express myself freely, and that the person on the end of the line will not shy away from me. I do not blame my friends – I would have behaved in the same way. I'm afraid until you've experienced it yourself, you don't have a clue what it's like … in that way, I'd say I am a more compassionate person now than I was before.

On my worst days, I would think of my grandsons in Canada who have lost their father. I would think yes, for my grandsons I must keep going … My son died eighteen months after my husband. To lose a spouse is one thing, but a child? How can there be a God? My son was forty-five years old, a children's doctor. He could save others, but he couldn't save himself.

Now, five years on, I am living a more 'normal' life. I don't have to leave the house every day. I accept the loneliness, it's not pleasant but it no longer terrifies me.

I force myself to try new things. At the grand age of sixty-odd I learned to swim and drive! I've even taken up bridge recently. Still, I sometimes feel socially isolated – like I'm in a no-man's land. I accept I fit with my new Cruse 'friends' only because we share a common bond in losing our partners. And though I still catch up with my old friends I don't really fit into their world anymore – so sometimes yes, I do feel out on a limb.

Past caring days are good and bad. If you know true love then you know true pain. Maybe that's what all this is about.

* * *

The 'void' was also a common theme amongst those folks partly past-caring. I call it 'partly past-caring' when a loved one is admitted to a home. This can be like bereavement.

Tracey, a thirty-year old woman from Cornwall, spent her late teens and most of her twenties caring. Because of a conflict within the family, Tracey took on the responsibility of looking after her grandmother who lived close-by. I ask her why. She says simply "I love my Grandma." Tracey was working and caring. It got too much. Her grandma, now 93, finally went into a home. Ten months later, I ask Tracey, what's life like?

Tracey's Story

It's the guilt that kills me. Grandma didn't want to go into a home, I let her down, I couldn't cope any longer. It's this exhaustion. You could sleep for a week and it doesn't go away. It penetrates your bones, your being. You can't get rid of it, this terrible, terrible tired.

It broke my heart when Grandma went into the home. But I've been ill myself, I was scared, what if I can't look after Grandma and she suffers? I'd hate that. And she was getting so poorly. The only person who didn't realise it was Grandma! I organised Home Care to come in to help get her up in the morning but she wouldn't let them in. I organised Meals On Wheels to call – but she wouldn't eat the meal. Stubborn? Oh, yes.

It put pressure on me but what do you do? I love her. I couldn't leave her lying there all day. So I'd go to Grandma's in the morning before work, get her up and organised, then, after work come by, wash her, do the house and get her ready for bed.

But when I wasn't there, she'd sit so close to the electric fire that she'd burn her legs. She was incontinent, her legs would get ulcerated, then infected. I'd sometimes go in and find her on the floor. I couldn't manage to lift her up so I'd have to phone an ambulance to come. I couldn't go on like that, I just couldn't cope. Social services finally got Grandma admitted to a home. I cried, even thought I knew it was for the best. Best doesn't make it easy, I couldn't help feeling guilty, like I was getting rid of her for my own needs. Truth is, I need Grandma as much as she needed me.

Her absence has highlighted how she had become the focus of my whole life. In my twenties I'd been too busy working and caring, I've never had a social life … so here I am, Miss Thirty and I'm suddenly free to go out and develop interests and hobbies and meet people, do whatever the hell I want when I want and it's such a shock that it feels scary.

After years of not having it, I now have time. I think, okay, what on earth am I going to do? And it's such a new thought the brain plays tricks.

After Grandma went into the home, I'd get back from work and think right, I'd better go up to Grandma's now... oh, I don't have to. I forgot to put Grandma's washing on... oh, I don't need to. I'd think, okay Tracey, watch telly. But even if it was a programme I'd usually have watched, now I'd be up pacing around the house ants-in-my-pants style. I'd think, okay, read. I'd get down a book I'd been meaning to read for ages only to find myself staring at the same page forever, the words just floating, no concentration. I'd think okay Tracey if not read, write … Yes, write a letter to a friend. But the letter wouldn't come together in any kind of coherent way. Someone actually wrote back, 'What the heck are you on about? Your letter just does not make sense, are you alright?'

I force myself to go out. I have a conversation with myself, a battle. Tracey go out, no, stay in, stay in, out, stay in, go out.

I go line-dancing once a week. It feels weird to be in a social environment. I feel guilty, like, I shouldn't be doing this, I shouldn't be here dancing away, I should be doing something constructive. I feel guilty for doing things and guilty for not doing things. I'm so used to doing things for everyone else, I can't get used to doing things for myself. I feel guilty about enjoying myself. But the truth is, I haven't enjoyed myself so much in years!

When I was a little girl I dreamt of being a paediatric nurse. Whilst caring for Grandma, I couldn't consider that career because it needed a big commitment and Grandma came first. What frightens me now is that I simply don't have the energy to re-train. Years of caring have left me drained. It feels like I once had a fire burning inside me and slowly but surely that fire has been extinguished until now there are only embers. I feel like I just haven't got the power to make the flame burn brightly again.

Exhausted. Burnt-out.

* * *

"I wish we were not so single-minded about keeping our lives moving, and for once could do nothing, perhaps a huge silence might interrupt this sadness of never understanding ourselves and of threatening ourselves with death."

Pablo Neruda

Memory: Twenty-eight years old

The rocking of the river was like a giant cradle. Inside the boat was dark, cosy, a protective womb. Outside the harsh February wind ruffled ducks and painted swirls in grey froth. From my bedroom window I could see swans being buffeted downstream, their slender necks twisted like hooks. The heavens were crying. Huge teardrops were flooding the park on the other side of the Thames. The footpath, usually bustling with parents, pushchairs, happy dogs, ambling old couples, is today deserted. I like it like that.

Like Garbo I want to be alone. Hide from the world, sleep, weep all day if it takes my fancy. I want to shrug responsibility, sip tea in bed 'til noon. I want to stop running and catch up with myself. I am choosing to drop out of the hurly-burly, remove myself from all pressure, all demands of any kind. I am treating myself to a year in retreat. I want No acting. No commitments. No expectations. No nothing. Just time for me.

My refuge is a houseboat called *Ondine*. Rented, but mine, alone. There are no neighbours, I don't know anyone in the town of Henley. This is what I want, need. Peace. Quiet.

The first night. I am awakened by the sound of knocking, urgent knocking. It is three o'clock in the morning but I am not sleeping. More in a twilight zone, mind racing, remembering, trying to forget. The urgent knocking makes me jump, my heart leap. I peer out into the darkness. Who is there? It comes again, rat-a-tat-tat. I duck under windows and slither on hands and knees to the far end of the boat. I fumble in drawers for a knife. The knocking comes in sporadic bursts, taunting. Because of the design, it is impossible to see who is at the door of my boat. I am scared but mad, furious, that someone should dare to disturb my new-found peace and quiet. I boldly fling open a window and swing myself out and clamber up, up, onto the flat roof of the boat. The air is nippy, my nightie barely existent. I brandish the knife before me like a toy dagger. The moon casts shadows as I circle, ready for combat. C'mon … c'mon, where are you? I am foolish and brave because I don't care anymore. Recently life has taken on an unreal, surreal feel, numbing. Is this really happening, I wonder. I'm not usually brave, usually I would have stayed indoors, called the police, emergency, come quickly, help. . I'm normally a scaredy-cat, so what am I doing miles from anywhere, no-one close enough to hear my cry for help? Like a wounded animal, I want to hide and once roused, attack. Rat-a-tat-tat … for God's sake, doesn't this nutter know why I am here? *Don't they know?* … "C'mon, c'mon", I yell to the void … yet only my shadow darts back and forth on the roof, with the river flowing and the boat rocking and the trees in the cool air whistling and there is no-one else here or there or anywhere.

The next day Jo, the girl who owned the boat, called by with her adorable two dogs. "Settling in?" she enquired kindly. I casually told her someone was knocking on my door at three in the morning. She smiled: "Swans". They peck the hull clean every night. "Sorry. I meant to tell you. Hope they didn't scare you?" "Not at all", I smile, thinking, I came to the country for peace and quiet and now I have a 3am swan-song!

We sip steaming tea crammed next to the only form of heating, a single calor stove. Jo knows why I am here. She shares with me that her dad is dead. I immediately warm to her, a kindred spirit. I cuddle the dogs; in the cold they make great fur coats.

"So, you're an actress," says Jo.

"Was," I correct her. "I'm taking time out."

"What are you going to do?"

"Nothing."

I was lucky to be in a position to do nothing. I appreciate not everyone can. There may be children to attend to, a husband or wife to still care for, a mortgage to pay.

I had a small amount of savings from work and I knew I would have some money coming once my parents' house was sold. This money I thought of as sad money, money I would rather never have had (I shed so many tears the day I received it.) But, in this period of utter burn-out, I was also immensely grateful for it. Thanks to my parents, I might now stop, rest, knowing at least, several months down the line, I would not end up in some cardboard box under Waterloo Bridge, as so many folk do when things collapse within them. Meanwhile, until that financial help came through, I signed on the dole and didn't look for a job. My improvising skills as an actress came in handy as I trekked fortnightly to sign my autograph.

"Miss Jenkinson, here's a job as a receptionist in a Steak House."

"Oh sorry, I can't, I'm vegetarian."

"Well you're not serving the food, simply seating people."

"No, no, the sight of it. I'd be sick, honestly, I'd be throwing-up over the customers."

"Well, here's a job in a pub."

"I … can't be around smoke. My sinuses get all swollen, like they're going to explode so's …"

"… here's office work …"

"Sorry, I have astigmatism in my left eye, if I look at a computer screen, it aches, so sore, the optician says to avoid …"

Ah, a reprieve for a fortnight.

On the way home I would celebrate surviving the Spanish Inquisition with a cappuccino and a bacon buttie. Any pangs of guilt about misuse of the tax-payers' money would be quashed because I knew. I knew that had I not been in the fortunate position to be able to 'stop', had I not followed my instinct and made the deliberate choice to rest, there was every chance, like an old car that has failed its MOT but continues to be driven by its jolly optimistic owner, that I would have ended up on some lonely road with something snapping, giving up, breaking-down. And I knew that would have cost the Government much more money to repair than the forty-odd quid a fortnight I received. If they could have repaired it, that is…

For the first year it was as if there was a veil between the world and me. I carried on functioning but I wasn't really there, if you know what I mean. I was running a Carers Support Group at the time. We'd meet weekly. Although I was concerned about all the individuals, in a sense, I wasn't the least bit interested in them. People used to say to me "Renee, after all these years, you've now got your freedom, you can go out, do things." But I couldn't have cared less about 'making a life' as it were. Perhaps it's nature's way of shielding you, protecting you for a while. I think there is something inherent in human nature that is resilient, and, after a period of time it says, I'm living, I've got to keep going, I've got to go shop … and you do. Like a natural fog slowly evaporates, I gradually began to emerge into a clearer state of being.

Renee, a carer for husband Bob for fourteen years after he suffered a stroke

I spoke to many carers who had been so exhausted for so long that when they stopped an avalanche of tiredness came crashing down. Many were so fatigued they did not know how they had filled the immediate void after the caring ended. They spoke of being in a mist, thick clouds, heads full of wool, limbs like lead, barely able to get out of bed, they spoke of negotiating this hectic world on automatic pilot. Over and over I heard the phrase, "I can't remember what I did right after."

For some the mist-like feeling may fade almost imperceptibly. For others there may be a defining moment that sees an increase in energy.

Over a coffee in a little café in the cobbled High Street of Edinburgh, Alan, 69, told me about Alice.

Alan's wife Alice suffered from Alzheimer's disease, a devastating disorder that destroys vital brain cells. A quantity surveyor, Alan took early retirement to care for Alice. Alan cared for Alice for fifteen years, seven of which Alice spent in long-term hospital care.

Alan's Story

For the first eighteen months after Alice died I can't tell you what I did. It's a blur. Sorry.

I met Alice when she was nineteen. She had beautiful red hair that later turned to gold, (and on occasions a temperament to go with it!) A bright and breezy personality, Alice was always fun to be with. We were very close, best friends.

After Alice died, I was lost. For so long I had followed the same routine, visiting the hospital twice a day. I liked to feed Alice. Although she could not speak, and we could no longer converse, deep in my heart I felt we still had contact with each other.

At around the age of fifty, things just started to go wrong. Alice was increasingly forgetful and began to have difficulty counting, reading, dressing. She was struggling to cope with her job as a Finance Assistant, had difficulties handling money.

… couldn't handle buses. Shopping.

She became agitated, depressed, weepy.

It took five years to get a diagnosis.

I was exhausted, on the go non-stop, got little or no sleep. My work was suffering. I organised a contact line to be linked directly to my office twenty miles away from home. I arranged a rota of willing bodies to care for Alice, her mother, friends, neighbours – but I often had to rush home as they found it difficult to cope.

I'll never forget the doctor's words. "It's incurable. There's nothing we can do for you."

We had both been looking forward to retirement, had made so many plans about what we'd do together, where we would go. Plans, dreams, never to be.

"It's incurable." I'll never forget those words.

On several occasions Alice asked me to give her an overdose. This was when she was still aware of her condition. She said it was "like being in a well, going further and further down and seeing the light disappear."

I couldn't do it. I was too much a coward. Not because I was afraid what might happen to me, but just making that decision, living through that moment of taking a life. I couldn't do it.

With Alice getting worse, I took early retirement. The day I retired I came back to an empty house. Alice was at day-centre. The silence was oppressive; Alice's presence, her light and laughter, gone.

Forty years of work and thirty-six years of marriage, both in a sense, come to an end. Waves of sadness swept over me.

The day Alice was finally admitted to long-term hospital care was like a death.

Gone forever. My Alice, taken from our house into long-term hospital care. It was the most traumatic decision of my life.

Home alone, I was restless. The things I used to enjoy, gardening, listening to music, no longer held any attraction. I couldn't concentrate. Half of me was elsewhere, with Alice.

My self-confidence plummeted. Since leaving work I had lost all social contact with the 'outside world'. I just didn't go out. I felt guilty that I couldn't do more for Alice and this led to a tendancy to deny myself any feelings of happiness or enjoyment.

More than once I sat by my wife's bedside, having being told she was not expected to 'make it'. I remember sitting by her bed and looking out the window and thinking how strange that the world keeps going on, that people are shopping and going to work and doing 'normal' things. I didn't feel a part of the world.

I was offered some freelance work as a surveyor in the construction industry. It would have meant working to ridiculous deadlines, being pushy and assertive at endless meetings, commuting to London. At one time this would have been appealing. Now it had lost its gloss. I turned it down.

At the hospital some relatives were invited to form a relaxation group. We were told we were 'carers'. That was a powerful moment. I'd never thought of it like that before. I was just a man looking after his wife.

Detached from the world, that's how I felt. In limbo.

More than the physical exhaustion was the emotional as daily I witnessed this ruthless disease robbing Alice of yet another function.

After Alice died I honestly can't tell you what I did.

I knew she had gone to a better place and would be warmly welcome there. I was glad … after so much suffering she was finally free.

Was I also free? Certainly I was relieved from my caring duties but I found it very strange not to have any hospital to go to, no Alice to visit. This had been my life for the last seven years.

Seven years.

The tiredness, all the years of resisting it, suddenly collapsed on me. Can't tell you what I did.

All I know is after eighteen months or so I booked a four-week holiday to Spain. Alice and I had been there several times. I went back to the same little mountain villages. Though at times, it was hard emotionally to be there, I felt a deep connection to Alice. I visited a small sleepy village where Alice and I had walked years before. In the village there was a shrine and little holes in the rocks where people could leave messages to their loved ones. I wrote a message to Alice and placed it into a crack in the rock. I then wandered across to a little outdoor café where I sat down and ordered a coffee. Within minutes, a white dove suddenly appeared out of the sky and flew down and landed right on the table next to me. It stared at me for a while, and I had an incredible sense of peace. There was a sense as if Alice was saying "it's okay, I am here. I am well. Everything is okay." Then it stretched its wings and flew away. Whatever it was, the sense of peace remained with me, and with it, I found an increase in my energy, both physical and mental.

Slowly, slowly I have regained my interest in gardening and listening to music. I also now do voluntary work with VOCAL (Voice of Carers Across Lothian) as I'm confident my experiences can help others. And at my daughter's insistence (Dad, you must do something that's not related to caring) I took up a new hobby, something I've always wanted to try my hand at – photography.

I'm sometimes asked if I feel angry at Alice's illness and the effect it had on us. It's not anger I feel but terrible sadness. Sadness that such a bright, sparkling person should have the best part of her life taken so cruelly. What does anger me is when I see people hurting each other, moaning and being petty about silly insignificant things. I feel like saying to them imagine somebody told you that very slowly, little by little, they are going to take away all your faculties, all your emotional and physical abilities until there's nothing left to take. Then you'd have something to moan about.

Memory: Twenty-eight years old

I can't abide the pettiness of people. I don't care for anyone. Hate everyone. Especially happy people. Worse; happy, successful people. And as for couples in love, well ... they make me want to puke.

One day my brother rang. He said, "Aunty Ann has had to have her leg cut off." I said "Why are you telling me?" "Because I thought you'd like to know," he said, sounding a bit stunned. "Oh well," I said. "Right. What's the weather like? Is it raining?"

It was great. This not-feeling feeling. Life just flowed over me. I bobbed along ... Everything was both important and trivial. I didn't mind if I died so long as I didn't suffer. I didn't matter. Nothing mattered. Emotional shutdown

I'm a mini-skirted party-girl, skinny-dipping in Henley mansion swimming-pools with people I barely know, people who are friends of friends of friends of the acquaintance I have come with.

Off to the regatta, all aboard, jumping on a stranger's boat, no idea whose, but a glass of champagne in my hand and ha, ha, ha.

Getting lifts, hitching, hi I'm Audrey, what's your name? ...

Blind-dates with Henley millionaires, Rolls-Royce waiting as I row across the flooded garden in a dinghy, tight black dress and wellies, struggling against the tide. Changing, like Cinderella, into silver strappy-sandals, depositing wellies in the mail-box, and off I'd go, purring into the night, cold bum on leather seat and champagne chilling, off to London to dine like a Queen, a sumptuous feast ... only to return emptier, emptier than before.

Having been accustomed to spending most of my life on the number 12 bus (I don't drive), there was, I admit, a certain thrill to being chauffeured around in a posh car, but it was all rather silly too. Having been accustomed to being in caring crisis situations (literally life or death moments), 'normal' life now seemed incredibly bland. Boring! Even though I was not living, for me, a 'normal' life. Having moved into a wealthy commuter belt, I suddenly found myself being invited to posh dinner parties by relative strangers. I went because I was doing nothing. Sitting in beautiful houses full of empty rooms far beyond the needs of the hosts would once have impressed me but now it seemed just plain daft. Why would people give up their life to work so they could afford a house much too big and three cars? It seemed ridiculous!

True, like a beggar, I'd had once pursued the image of success. Believed that when I got this or that, then I would be happy. Always chasing the future. I'd seen too many sexy adverts, skimmed too many glossy magazines and compared myself too much with those in them. I had believed, along with others, what made-up the hallmarks of a 'successful' life. "What do you do?" I'd ask someone and cast my judgement.

"What do you do Audrey?"

"Nothing."

"… What would you like to do?"

"Nothing."

Silence. The host and fellow-guests, usually an array of professionals, would stare in disbelief. (I learned it was very difficult to live in the world and do or want nothing. Nobody believed you!)

"You can't do nothing!"

I would feel the need to explain. To justify?

"Well, I was helping look after my Mum and she died and … well, I'm so tired…"

"How long ago was that?"

"About six months now…" Six months sounded ages ago. Like I should be up and running again by now.

"My taxes are keeping you." It would be said as a joke. "Wish I could lie in bed all day." I'd make the mistake of getting entangled in defending myself. I'd try to explain more about this state of being, the aftermath of caring … But I couldn't describe it. Couldn't find the words.

"Thought you were an actress," my hosts would say. "Bet you wouldn't turn down De Niro if he called up."

"Would too. I'd tell him sorry Bob, I'm resting."

It was the truth but it sounded unbelievable. Ever since I could remember I had wanted to be an actress. Yet now, if I had been offered the lead in the best script ever, I would have turned it down. There was no longer any emotion within to draw upon. No longer any sense of excitement, of passion, for acting. For anything. It appeared not only had I lost my parents, but myself. I had always been someone who followed my heart and now my heart rattled around in my chest. Empty.

In the light of what had happened, the world of acting now seemed too fake. I had seen behind the scenes. Knew how we were touched-up. Knew how the media manufactured fairytale lives. Hadn't I read about myself in print and thought gosh, I'd like to be her!

So many illusions killed by illness, shattered by death. What once seemed so important, is now too worthless. I thought, I play a few good parts and then I die? So what? Now it made me sick how much money and pampering actors got for just pretending. What about carers? How much did they get for dealing with reality?

I gave away my telly. Utter rubbish. Stopped reading glossy magazines. Waste of precious time.

Society had got it wrong. It rewarded trivia.

"But Audrey, don't you want to be successful?" my dinner party friends persisted.

I told them, not in an arrogant way, that I thought I already was. I told them I thought caring for someone until they die is a success. It's just a shame it's not recognised as such. Not up there alongside a supermodel showing off a dress or a footballer scoring goals or being the chairman of a corporate company. They looked at me as if I had lost my marbles.

I could understand it. In our society, it is rare to consider the woman or man down the road caring for a husband or wife as doing something amazing. As some kind of hero or heroine. I too certainly would never have considered it like that before I had experienced the illness and deaths of my parents.

I could also understand my dinner friends' lack of understanding my wanting nothing. In life, it is rare we ever get, or are brave enough to take, an opportunity to stop running. There is a fear of getting left behind, missing out …

… because every time we walk down the street, switch on the television, we are told we need something. If only we buy this, get that, we will be complete.

As I walked into Henley to get my coffee in the morning, I would see lots of flashy cars, tired harassed occupants on mobile phones, and I would recall a pet saying of my Dad's. Usually after a wee dram he would raise his eyebrows and ask in a quizzical tone "What's it all about? Mmm. What's it all about?"

And I'd walk past thinking, poor souls, don't they know? Don't they know with the flick of a pinkie it all comes crashing down?

For as if blasted out of a sleep-walk, now I know. I know there is no acting part big enough, no riches abundant enough, no fame elaborate enough that could, would make any difference. For who cares about career, about money, status, power, people even when now I know . . . nothing can fill this emptiness. I have spent my life forever wanting, aching with want. Now I want nothing. And in wanting nothing, I have never known such freedom.

I stare out at the world from Noah's Ark and wonder . . has the world capsized or have I?

The Portuguese call it *saudade,* which translates as a deep yearning, an inexplicable longing in the soul. I consciously desired nothing, yet there was a churning in my guts that made me restless. It seemed that, in the wake of my parents' deaths, I must find something real for my life. Something that mattered. The paradox was this. If nothing can make a difference, then surely nothing matters?

I struggled with this ... precariously swinging from one tree of thought to the next – if death takes all, if nothing lasts, why begin anything? You work hard to achieve a goal but when you get there it's meaningless. Love too gets taken, snatched from within your arms in the dead of night. Or one day it leaves, willingly, whoosh, out the door, gone. The books I was reading at the time talked about this impermanence, how nothing in life is secure even when we like to think it is. They talked of the importance of seeing this in relation to life, to death. Buddhists referred to it as 'non-attachment'. Well what's the point of starting anything, I thought, just skip straight to end, save yourself time, effort and heartache. I became attached to non-attachment.

...But ... if I should die today, tomorrow, next year or in forty, I don't want to look back and think ...

... I wasted my life.

So the dilemma is: how can I live a meaningful life when I believe in nothing? When everything seems pointless. Unreal.

I looked around, searched ...

In splendid country houses, pleasant couples would entertain, cute kids run riot and warm fires blaze, and I'd think, maybe they have the secret, maybe they have something real - but then the illusion is shattered as the lady of the house goes to fetch something and the gentleman discreetly asks for my number. I refuse.

Dinner with a friend, a businessman, who is treating two clients over from America. He is charming, the perfect host, telling them how wonderful it has been to have them here, how much he has enjoyed it, how he can't wait' til next time, what a joy, what a pleasure it's been to see them. As we bid goodnight and climb into shiny metal, he tells me how he can't stand them, what a pain, thank God the Yanks are fucking off home. He is an extremely successful businessman. Leading a schizophrenic life. Is it worth it? I ask him. You have to play the game, he replies.

I searched …

… and the more I searched the more I came to know the deep dissatisfaction that lay within a wealth of happy faces.

I began to ask why? Past caring, life was urgent. Forget some day, one day: what about today? We could fall down, overboard, at any moment. So why spend precious time pretending?

I began to ask people, if you hate your wife why don't you leave? Why do you work so hard, why? Are you fulfilled? Inspired? If you had six months to live, what would you be doing? So why aren't you doing it? Yes, you may have all this and that but what do you dream of in the far reaches of the night? What regrets will visit you on your deathbed? So why are you wasting so much time and energy on petty tittle-tattle? Why?

Being an orphan brought with it a sense of headiness, of rebellion: not you or you or you can tell me what to do because only my parents can and I am parent-less.

I became outspoken, challenging, a liability to have around at those posh dinner parties.

I had a need, a longing to expose, to strip everything away. All the bullshit. All the masks, the hypocrisy, the endless smokescreens, uncover them to get to the core of what was real.

I see now … it was not others but myself I was trying to understand.

And I see now … even when I thought I was doing nothing, something was happening. Despite the old ground falling away, leaving me with the feeling of dangling on some tightrope heaving with opposing thoughts, if we can just hang on, … watch, listen, trust … maybe, far below, out of sight in the darkness, a new seed will take root. Begin to grow.

> **Care Fact**
> Research indicates that there could be anywhere between
> 19,000–51,000 young people who undertake being the main
> carer in the home. It is very difficult to know the exact number
> because of the hidden nature of the caring.

I asked a group of able-bodied healthy people who had had no experience of caring to look back on their teenage years and tell me what they would have missed most if they had had to care for an ill parent on a full-time basis:

- Working, I began work at seventeen as a library assistant, it felt great to be grown-up, earning money.
- Going to the dancing, a great big group of us, what a laugh.
- Getting stoned.
- University, though I got kicked out after twelve months!
- Visits to the cinema, Paul Newman ...
- Seeing friends when I wanted to, whenever I wanted to.
- Travelling – I hitch-hiked across Afghanistan, through the Kyber Pass, on into India. Incredible! Worth any amount of Delhi-belly.
- Art school – I was middle-class, art school drew me out, liberated me ...
- Late nights out and late lie-ins.
- Sex – not having to rush home in the morning ... unless I wanted to, of course.
- Independence day! – Moving into my first ever flat.
- Drumming – learning drums, forming a band, first gigs! Leaving Belfast for a contract in London. Yeh, I probably wouldn't be a drummer today.
- Following the love of my life to Australia – we've now been happily married thirteen years.
- Getting drunk, partying.
- Just being able to go out with my mates ...

The following comments are based on many interviews with carers. I let the voices bleed into one:

– We're angry. We're pissed off. We're just past caring.

– What do you mean the computer can't accept my circumstances? I'm not fit for work. No, I'm not disabled. Just past caring.

– I'm 55 years old. I cared for twelve years. I live per week on what most couples spend in one go at Tesco.

– Look I really would like this job. Oh … you want to know how I'll manage to get up in the morning after so many years out of the workplace? You're worried that I'll not be on time in the morning? … I want to scream: Look, you daft numptie, I've been getting up three times during the night for the last thirty years to turn and toilet my incontinent and physically deformed mother, for the last thirty years I've been up at six-thirty every morning to make sure I eat breakfast because I don't know if I'll have a chance to eat again, depending on how that particular day goes, no two days being the same, and I was up to give Mum her breakfast at eight, every morning for thirty years, so please don't be concerned, don't be worried if I can get to work on time for nine. But I want the job, am desperate for the job, so I smile and say, "Oh getting up shouldn't be a problem". I don't get the job. I don't get any job.

– They found a gap in my NHI contributions. Nine years. From childhood to age forty-three, I was sole carer for my helpless Mum. I missed only nine years. They took 12% off my state retirement pension. Over £500 p.a. A lot when you're 82. I approached Isle of Man DHSS with a proposition: Abolish the contributions principle for people who have been carers. They never replied.

– "So what are you going to do now?" Stop, stop asking questions, please stop, I want to talk. I need to talk. Just … listen.

– We don't want plaudits. We need practical support. Practical support not pleasant words.

– I'm now agoraphobic. It could be something to do with hardly leaving the house in eighteen years as sole carer for my wife. No, I can't just pop down. . I'm afraid I can't pop anywhere.

– I had been a 'jobseeker' for six months and they were putting pressure on me to find a job and I was trying to sell the house because I could not afford the upkeep on my own and I was dealing with all the grief, bereavement, the years of caring and the pressure just got too much, too much and I had a sort of mini-breakdown. I'm now on the sick with 'stress'. But I'm scared they'll put the pressure on again …

– Some days I felt it was humanly impossible to go on any longer, but somehow I did. I have no idea how I did… (*Monica, a carer*)

* * *

Carers keep going because they have to. They lurch from one crisis to the next, endless days and nights with no respite, no time for self. Parents of small children may go through a similar process of neglecting their own needs to fulfil those of another. The sleep deprivation may be similar, the exhaustion, the loss of your own freedom to do what you like, when. But ultimately, the caring for a healthy growing child, although demanding, is not as draining on the soul as caring for someone in pain; watching them waste away, suffer, die. The physical wear and tear on muscles and limbs as a carer struggles to lift, bathe, to dress a dependent adult differs from the manoeuvring of a spirited toddler into his tracksuit.

Adrenaline becomes the reliable friend of the carer, zapping pain into submission, numbing emotions to enable them to cope, keep going.

When caring stops, a floodgate opens. Aches, both emotional and physical, can now safely surface. I heard stories, lots …

   – Slipped discs, muscle spasms, sciatica
   – Depression, chronic fatigue, social phobia, anxiety
   – Addicted to tranquillizers, sleeping pills
   – Break-ups and break-downs
   – Migraines, high blood pressure
   – Stress, colds, fevers, flu that doesn't go
   – Eczema, acne, puss-filled boils, shingles
   – Suicidal thoughts, psoriasis, dandruff
   – Periods that start. Stop. Zig-zag, all over the place
   – Panic attacks. Sweating, clammy, dizzy, disorientated. The world slowing down, heart racing, palpitating. Feeling so ill, so faint …

Maggie, a single mother of two children and a carer for her parents, tells me: "As my children grew out of nappies my mother grew into them." She recalls her experience of a panic attack on her first day out after her mother's funeral:

I'm sitting on the bus, heading into Cambridge town centre, looking forward to a wander round the shops. Sitting on the bus, one minute feeling fine, then suddenly all funny, faint, shaky; scared I'm going to pass out, have to get off, get off the bus, quickly. See a church, thank God, a little café inside. In I go, all wibbly-wobbly. The staff, so kind, so understanding, sit me down, take good care of me, tell me I will be okay, but I am scared – what is happening?

The doctor tells me it's a panic attack. A moment and then it hits me. The rare occasions I'd go out when Mum was alive I'd first have to arrange a 'Mum-sitter', going out could not be spontaneous but had to be planned, always I would arrange to go out somewhere with a friend. A shocking realisation. I have not been further than our local post office just down the street on my own in years. I am forty-four years old and can't travel into town on my own!

Determined to beat the problem, I made a point of catching the same bus daily, always heading to the safety of the little café where I knew the staff would understand. I kept a diary of feelings, sensations, of how far I got or didn't get that particular day. Gradually, I was able to venture further into the hustle, bustle, knowing I could go back to the café, my anchor-point, should I feel 'funny'. Finally, a triumph. I managed to enter the town centre and go to the shops on my own! But only small shops, big stores like Debenhams were out of bounds. I didn't have much money so small charity shops suited me fine. Today, five years on, I still can't cope with large stores or supermarkets.

Graham tells me how caring damaged his health:

"After my wife died people said 'She's at rest now. You must live your own life now.' 'Join a club Graham,' they said. 'That'll give you something to do.' There were fitness clubs, cricket clubs, football and badminton and happy-clappy clubs for folks much older than me. I'm not old but I feel old. I'm now feeling all the aches and pains I've ignored over the years. The doctor says be careful, take it easy but it's not easy. What to do? I suppose there's always the Women's Institute line dancing."

Grief and Guilt

Grief

On the heels of the physical and mental burn-out prevalent to past caring comes grief. Grief normally follows the death of a loved one in any circumstances, whether involved in caring for them or not. Individuals experience the pain of grief in their own unique way. But, in the melting pot of emotions, past carers spoke to me, wrote to me, of one emotion that bubbled up again and again.

Guilt

There were times when I had this feeling of anger and hatred towards her when she was alive. I loved her but sometimes I was just so stressed trying to cope with everything and I'm afraid I took it out on her. After she died came the overwhelming guilt. I had a very helpful GP who I could talk to. I think it's important to ask for help. Now I've learned to say I did the best I could at the time. And I did. I did the best I could at the time.

(Sophie, a carer for her mother for eighteen years)

I felt guilty I hadn't been more loving. As a carer I was so exhausted I operated on automatic pilot. I wish I'd had more energy to be loving.

(Keith, a carer for his wife for fourteen years)

I felt guilty because he died in a nursing home when I can clearly remember telling him I would always look after him at home. After his death a thought haunted me. Could I have kept him at home longer? I felt a lot of guilt over not knowing how much he was aware of in his last few months and at times getting impatient with him. Guilty of the feelings of just wanting to give up and put the caring in someone else's hands.

(Shirley, a carer for her husband)

The council installed a flue outside our kitchen wall that meant fumes blew directly into our house. David's emphysema had definitely got worse after that. I felt like I'd really let David down. I was full of anger and guilt at the council, at myself. Could I have done more?

(Margaret, a carer for husband, David)

After my mother died my youngest (of four children) was following me around like a limpet. She wouldn't let me out her sight, was always getting 'round my feet', I began to think what's wrong with her? Then I realised. Every day after school she would go in and sit on the bed and tell her Grandma about her day. As a busy Mum, helping my husband with a business that we ran from home and caring for my own Mum, I had little time to listen to her because I was always on the go. I realised that she was missing Grandma. I felt so guilty! From then on I made a concerted effort to make time for my youngest daughter, to sit down with her and really listen to what she was saying.

(Betty, Reading)

I am Muslim. I'm not a practising Muslim but after dad died I began to get up at dawn to pray. I began to wear a black scarf over my head. It was out of guilt. I felt that if I didn't something awful might happen to Dad's soul.

(Carina)

I felt guilty and angry because when she went into the Home and began to be cared for there, it was like okay, you've done your bit, now we're taking over. I felt excluded, even though I knew best what Mum needed. I felt bad. Like Mum would think I had abandoned her.

(Frank, a carer for his Mum with Alzheimer's)

I had not had a holiday in ten years. At my son's insistence I went away on holiday and when I came back mother was dying. I felt so guilty. But if I hadn't had the holiday I don't think I could have coped with her dying.

(Maggie)

* * *

Grief brings up not only guilt but loss. Denial. Regret. Sadness. Anger. Relief … and more guilt at feeling relief. When caring stops a sea of strange emotions, both new and buried, now floats to the surface, rising, falling, now stormy, now calm. Unpredictable, these waves sweep us into uncharted waters. We toss this way and that, now fine, sick, fine and yet sick again.

Past carers spoke of grief not only for their loved one, but themselves. For the years that had passed since their life got interrupted, put on hold. Anger and grief for all that they had missed out on. Sadness and grief for what could have been.

Some spoke of anger now directed at others. They felt raw and sore that all the caring had been left down to them. They felt burdened and abandoned. They spoke of fall-outs within families and never forgiving.

Some people spoke of feeling so bereft there was a feeling of what's the point? My loved one has gone. I don't care anymore.

After Dad died, there was no reason to get up in the morning. Nobody needed me. I would go to bed praying that I wouldn't wake up. To build a new life seemed such an effort. I hardly ate, smoked like a chimney, veged in front of the telly, drank beer. I couldn't care about me one iota. I got awful colds. I couldn't be bothered with Vitamin C. Just had another cigarette.

(Alan, Newcastle)

Grief plunges us into a world where nothing seems secure. It can be a frightening chaotic place where we struggle to stay afloat.

It is important, during this vulnerable time, to be supported mentally, physically and spiritually. It is important to ensure that you give yourself as much self-care as possible.

For people past caring it can feel strange to have the time to nurture their own health. So strange that some past carers told me they had forgotten how to care for themselves, it felt odd, selfish, they told me they felt guilty, like they didn't deserve it.

I have a dream … there is a rambling house in the Border valleys of Scotland, it is called 'The Welcome Rest'. It is set in rolling lawns through which a small river winds. Rabbits dart wild round purple Rhododendron. Inside log fires burn in rooms furnished in warm, vibrant colours with flannel sheets and soft pillows. There is a library with comfy sofas and walls packed with inspirational books. There is a kitchen where a cook prepares home-grown nutritious food for the guests. Meals are served in a light dining room where guests can eat alone or with others and nobody judges. There are small therapy rooms where guests can have massage, counselling, acupuncture. How much or little you do here is up to you. You can walk in the hills or lie before the fire. You can wail or laugh. However you want to be here you are welcome. It doesn't cost anything to come here but if you can afford it, donations are always appreciated. They will help others who wish to come here to experience a taste of what it is to be cared for. It is a safe place, supportive. Rest-full.

I would love to see a place like this. It is desperately needed, long overdue. Again and again I heard stories of how past carers longed for a place to go to be supported in their journey from carers back into mainstream society. Ursula suggested a place like this could act as a bridge, to absorb the shock between caring and past caring.

So many carers long to stop, rest, to have space to grieve but can't due to financial or domestic circumstances.

Carers who have young children have no choice but to keep going. They may have been caring for an ill husband or wife and now they wish they could lie in bed and pull the covers over their head but little voices are calling for breakfast, a school shirt to be ironed, a lift to a friend's house. You get up, put on a cheery smile and carry on.

In that respect, children can be a lifeline. James, forty-four, is one of many carers who says: "Had it not been for the little life that now relied on me so totally for survival I would have simply given-up on the world. There would have been no purpose to my life."

His story is one of the most bitter-sweet I have ever heard:

James' Story

We were both forty-two. We'd been married thirteen years. We had a good marriage, very loving. We'd delayed starting a family so we could spend time together. We'd done a lot of travelling, both had careers, we had some financial security and decided the time was ripe to try for a family. We were very lucky, Elaine fell pregnant almost immediately. We were overjoyed! Several weeks later, though, our joy turned to panic. Elaine had discovered a nasty lump on her breast. It turned out to be a malignant tumour. Because of the type of cancer it was, they couldn't operate right away. The doctors compared it to a dandelion flower – if disturbed the spores would immediately scatter and spread into the bloodstream. The hospital told us they could offer chemotherapy. If we did not want to lose the baby we would have to wait until Elaine was sixteen weeks or so into her pregnancy. Or they could abort the baby and begin now. The course of chemotherapy meant that Elaine could not fall pregnant in the future. Should she survive, that is. Nobody knew if she would, but the hospital said they thought her chances were better if she discontinued with the pregnancy. We were given a few days to think about it. The hospital said they would support us in whatever decision we made. After much discussion and sleepless nights agonising over what to do, we made our decision. We would go ahead with the pregnancy. Elaine decided it was a risk worth taking. There was no guarantee that she would live even with an abortion and earlier treatment. And so, at the minimum safe term of pregnancy, she began a course of six chemotherapy treatments. Each time, they would do a scan to make sure the baby was okay. After the fifth scan the baby wasn't moving. Elaine was rushed in for an emergency caesarean at seven and a half months. Baby Edward, who weighed 2lbs went straight into intensive care. Elaine stayed in hospital for a while and was given a final dose of chemotherapy. That dose made her terribly ill, as she was already weakened by the operation. Edward was six weeks old, now weighing 4lbs and still in Intensive Care when doctors made the decision to operate on Elaine. They said the tumour had shrunk sufficiently to do so. Elaine went in for a mastectomy. I raced between two hospitals, one where Edward lay battling for life, the other where Elaine lay battling for life, as well as finding the energy to will on her little son to survive.

I work in publishing and lumped every holiday together to have time off. It was a nightmare time. Hell. Words cannot describe it.

To my delight, in the November, I got both my wife and son home. The mastectomy appeared to have been a success. We had been given a special food formula to help build Edward up. Things were looking up. Edward needed a lot of care as did Elaine but she managed to feed him sometimes and she loved to hold him and kiss him and play with him. He was still tiny but to us, he was perfect. He was ours. For the first time in ages I dared to dream of a future with my family. I thought everything was going to be okay.

Then, over Christmas, Elaine caught what she thought was a terrible cold. She was dizzy and her ears ached. Her GP gave her antibiotics but they did no good. She got weaker. The hospital told her to come in for a treatment of radiotherapy just in-case ... and it was then they discovered ... the cancer had spread to her brain. There was nothing anyone could do. She spent time at home and, as things got worse, she was admitted to hospital. Her brother helped take care of her there, sleeping over in her room. I visited with Edward every day. She loved to see him. To see how each day he was growing bigger, stronger.

Elaine died on Mother's Day, 10 March, 2002.

Edward has been my lifeline. I am too busy attending to his every need I have no time to feel sorry for myself. Every hour he's demanding something. He's sixteen months now. All he's interested in is food, milk, sleep and hugs. Oh yes, and a clean nappy.

Edward goes to a child-minder across the street when I go to work. I drop him off at 8.30am and pick him up at 3.30pm. I don't take any breaks and work right through my lunch-hour so I can leave early to pick him up. He still wakes during the night, but he's getting better.

I have no regrets about the decision we made. It would have been unbearable if we had aborted the baby and Elaine had died too. Any way we turned was a risk, a gamble. What is a miracle is that Edward survived at all. I have lost someone precious but I have gained someone precious. I look upon Edward as a gift. He is Elaine's gift to me. Part of her lives on in him. And one day, when he's old enough, I'll sit down with my son and tell him all about his brave, beautiful mother.

* * *

A parent carer who has been caring for a spouse deals not only with their own grief but also the grief of the children. This can be a very healing experience for everyone if handled sensitively.* But the tendency may be for the parent to focus exclusively on the child and in so doing deny themselves much-needed 'down' time.

Grief may then emerge at a much later date. The body has a way of saying okay, it's 'safe' for these feelings to come out now. Often it is not until we stop running around and have some down-time that we can truly begin to feel what is going on for us inside. If we have been ignoring, or avoiding painful feelings, they do not go away. They just get pushed deeper down inside us. No wonder then it can feel scary to stop.

Shonagh had no children to 'keep going' for but rather found keeping ultra-busy acted as a distraction. Although Shonagh wasn't aware of it at the time, keeping busy for her meant there was no time to think. To *feel.*

---

* Winston's Wish is a charity that provides support for bereaved children and the relatives of a bereaved child.

"I kept going so I wouldn't have to deal with the previous five years of hell, so much illness, death, so much repressed anger inside me, grief for the young woman who felt robbed of her twenties, robbed of a healthy mother, a mother who, because of illness, wasn't able to give her daughter the support to help her grow, blossom into a well-balanced young woman. I just didn't want to face this explosive cocktail of feelings. I was afraid to."

Shonagh (33)

Though Shonagh had a severe flu that would not leave her, she described the first year after her mother's death as 'living at a hundred miles an hour, filling every single moment'. She didn't stop – until she had to!

Shonagh's Story

I was thirty years old. After years of being ill with MS, Mum was dead. I had a terrible flu but was determined to keep busy. I pushed myself and got a job working back in pharmacology, a job that involved lots of travelling, catching early flights to Amsterdam. I was exhausted but kept going, just numbed myself to everything including this terrible flu.

When I was a child my little sister told me in a hushed whisper that Mum had fallen down the stairs. I wasn't to tell anyone. Everything in our family was shrouded in secrecy. Our Mum walked with a stick, she couldn't do things other Mums could do but nobody explained why to us children. Mum was often short-tempered. Looking back I see it was to do with her dealing with the MS but no-one told us about it. In a way it was denial. We sensed something was wrong but everyone acted as if everything was fine.

When I was fourteen, things at home were not good. Mum's illness was progressing but we didn't discuss it. I got very depressed and threw myself into my schoolwork as a way of deflecting it. I drove myself hard with my studies, put on a happy face and kept myself really busy. This pattern continued to university. Studying madly, going out lots, drinking lots, throwing myself obsessively into all kinds of sports; keeping busy was a great way to avoid thinking about everything.

Age twenty-five I was working as a pharmacologist for a major drugs company in Windsor. The pattern continued, the crazy life, working like a Trojan, travelling lots, socialising lots, partying late, then racing back to spend weekends helping with Mum (Dad was the main carer) then up Monday morning to catch the 6 a.m. flight back to London, straight to work, socialising after work, running on sheer adrenaline, when boom …

Age twenty-nine, and after four years of this hectic lifestyle, I wasn't coping. I couldn't cope with the workload and Mum's illness. I quit my job. I could cut the ties with Windsor. I couldn't cut the ties with my Mum.

The day I left Windsor, I shut the door on my life there. Just blocked off the man I had been going out with for about a year. I felt so bad about myself. Felt I had nothing to offer him, felt my life wasn't going anywhere. I isolated myself. It seemed the Windsor crowd could not relate to what it was like to juggle a demanding career and an ill mother.

I came back to Edinburgh and got a job in a pub. I was drinking a lot, sort of drowning everything out. Mum was between home and respite. I resented her being ill. I wanted to be free, like my friends, to build my life without having to race back every two minutes to face this nightmare situation.

What I didn't see then, that I see now, is that I could have had a healthy, fulfilling life in Edinburgh with caring for Mum being a part of that life. I could have had a good career in Edinburgh and still have been able to help with Mum. Unfortunately, at that time I thought I could only 'have a life' if I went elsewhere. So I bolted abroad.

I applied to teach English in Japan. When I got accepted I remember thinking, oh I have to go now, the ball is rolling. I see that by telling myself I had no choice, it assuaged any guilt.

When I left Edinburgh, I didn't feel anything. It seemed the only way I could cope with everything was to switch off emotionally and mentally. Numb out. That's the only way I could exist.

Japan was a complete release. I enjoyed the work and began to regain some confidence. Then, four months into a year contract, I got news that Mum was due to go in to hospital for a routine operation. Dad said don't come back, stay. I thought oh God, should I stay or should I go? It was hellish, I was a total stress-bucket. Mum's illness had been going on for years, since I was a child, really, and I knew it could go on for years to come. I decided to stay, then thought no, it doesn't feel right. I managed to get a flight back on the day Mum was having her operation.

I got into Heathrow in the evening and called home to let them know that I had arrived. Dad told me that Mum was dead. She had died earlier that day, as I was flying home.

I wanted to howl with rage. Just as I had taken a step to get my own life back on track I had lost her.

I had terrible feelings of guilt. It took me two years and much counselling to come to the realisation that I was only away for four months and that I had spent the previous five years racing back and forth.

A few weeks after the funeral, I returned to Japan. I wasn't thinking straight, I didn't know what else to do. I went back. Back to the manic lifestyle, keeping ultra-busy, I came down with a terrible flu. I was miserable. I felt like I didn't belong there anymore. Ironically, now I was completely free to stay I didn't want to be there. I packed my bags and came home.

I lived with Dad. Nothing could shift this terrible flu. I got a job back in pharmacology, a job that again meant demands, pressure, lots of travelling, catching early flights to Amsterdam. This terrible flu wouldn't leave me. I was exhausted but ignored it, just kept going, on and on, like in some kind of shock, just going through the motions, living at 100 miles an hour on and on and on and …

STOP

I couldn't get out of bed. My body had completely given up on me. Not a shred of energy, not a drop of reserve in the tank. Just physical, emotional and mental burn-out. Breakdown.

By this time I had bought my own flat and was living on my own. It had been a year since my mother had died. I had kept going so I wouldn't have to deal with the previous five years of hell. So much suppressed anger boiling inside me.

I slid into clinical depression, barely ate. Just going down, down … didn't trust anyone … gave up on life … lost confidence, lost myself … feeling utterly worthless. I wanted to pack a bag and go live on the streets. I felt I didn't belong anywhere.

The Windsor crowd were caught up in career, making money and babies, how could they relate to what I'd been through? I realised some so-called 'friends', well, they were nice people but there was no real point of contact between us. I'd had all this burden of experience and I felt my friends didn't have a clue. Yes, one friend stuck by me and she had no experience of long-term caring but I needed someone to say "Look, I know what you've been through. I looked after my Mum or Dad, yes, I know, I know …"

I knew nothing of carer groups at that time. I wish I had. I wish that, when I was a teenager, I'd have been able to go to a young carers group. But if a parent doesn't acknowledge an illness, doesn't accept it, how can a child?

The depression lasted two years.

You couldn't call this time 'living.' I existed. I slept a lot, just managed to the shops to get food. I was diagnosed with ME. After everything with Mum, it was as if I'd said okay, now it's my turn to get ill. Whilst Mum was alive I'd kept going. When she died, and I was free to pursue my life, I simply stopped functioning.

This cocktail of emotions was potent. Yes, Mum's death was a relief, but with the relief came guilt. Rage at what had happened to her and to me, to my life over the years. Sadness that she was gone mixed with strange elation at being free. It felt odd that I could now do what I wanted. This liberation was scary, hard to adjust to. It had been easier for me to be the people-pleaser.

During this time of the depression I was having vivid disturbing dreams, in every one of them I was always fifteen years old. It was as if, subconsciously, I never got beyond being a teenager, never was able to cut the ties of my Mum's needs to become my own person.

Fears rose up, fear of getting ill myself. I'd think, what's the point of starting something new because I may get ill or others may get ill and I'll have to look after them. This constant fear of getting MS crippled me emotionally.

I sought alternative healing, exploring everything from Chinese medicine to homeopathy.

There was a Christian Fellowship of Healing down the street from my house. One day I decided to go in for a healing session. It was very gentle, like a laying on of hands. Afterwards I felt better, calmer. I went back several times. The healers were very caring. I became interested in going to church. I was seeking something, didn't quite know what … then somebody lent me some Christian tapes by Liberty Savage. I listened to them every day. Within two weeks the severe depression started to lift. It was incredible. I began to feel so much better about myself, about life. I thought, okay, I have to get back out there. But where to start?

I have to take things slowly because I still have ME. At the moment I'm doing voluntary work at the local carers centre. Mostly the carers are older but I feel comfortable with them, they are more understanding than people my own age.

Social-life wise, I haven't had a boyfriend for ages. I suppose I don't easily let men in. When grieving, sometimes pure raw emotions come out of nowhere. You don't know what will happen next. Unless you've been there, it's hard to understand or offer real support. One male friend admitted very honestly, "I've never lost a parent so I don't know what to say."

A lot of my peers haven't had to deal with a parent's illness and dying. And it reverberates so deeply it's hard to open up, to get close to someone.

Now I'm feeling better, I see that it's absolutely okay to be single. I now revel in my independence. Perhaps one day I'll meet a good man and have children but I'm not ready for children yet. I'm enjoying doing things for me just now.

I recently helped organise a creative day for the Ministry of Healing. It's wonderful to be creative, whether it's woodwork or pottery or doing the garden. Even if you make something tiny, it makes your soul feel better. Before I would have had ideas but never had the confidence to see it through. Now I love the process of realising the vision. It's huge, when you realise the power of your own creativity. Very healing.

I am currently doing a course for re-training in computers. I'm also interested in training as an alternative health-care practitioner, perhaps a Shiatsu therapist. I would like to be able to help people in a way that empowers them to help themselves. I don't want to care for anyone who is totally reliant ever again.

I'm learning to care for me, to build up boundaries. To say no. It has taken me two years to realise I'm not going to look after my Dad. He said to me, "If I fall ill you'll have to look after me." I said, "No I won't. I want to be a daughter, not a carer."

One year on from the depression I am now on the cusp of a new life. I see I have choices.

Before the breakdown I would have thought of being 'successful' in terms of business; running your own business, making money, showing profit, doing well. Or being good at your job, people having a high opinion of you, to be a 'somebody' in the workplace.

Now, for me, success means a good healthy positive relationship with yourself and others, being able to say no, being able to express your needs and ask for help and going after your dreams and desires where possible. Now I want to be successful for me, live my life for me, rather than to impress others or fit-in with other people's perceptions or expectations of me.

Some of my old Windsor friends are driving around in their BMWs earning ridiculous salaries and eating in the best restaurants but they never see their children. Both partners work, they have nannies that are basically surrogate parents.

I look at them and think that could've been me, I had that kind of job, I know how easy it is to get caught up in the rat-race. But would I have found that life fulfilling? Certainly, for me now, having been through what I have, material things hold no value, what people have materially is of no consequence. What matters more to me is that someone is a good person, not personality but character, that they are honest, reliable, trustworthy, caring, compassionate.

Life is simpler, yet more rewarding now. Before I was working too hard, moving too fast, never being satisfied with my life. I'm learning now to appreciate each moment. In this period of stillness, good memories have come up too. I look back on my life and think, why didn't I appreciate, why didn't I enjoy that time more? I'm determined not to make the same mistake. A saying I find very inspiring is 'The opportunity of a lifetime should be taken in the lifetime of the opportunity.'

I am now more aware of myself, of others, of what I am doing, of how I feel. I'm more in the present. I appreciate more the people I am with. I notice things around me like I never did before. I see God at work everywhere. Just seeing a flower fills me with joy.
Sometimes I look back and think; perhaps I needed the breakdown to bring me to this new place?

I asked other past carers, what helped them in their voyage of discovery to bring them to new places:

Counselling

- Through counselling, I've recognised that the rage inside me was actually not anger but pain. Pain at watching how my wife suffered, I helpless to change things. I had this anger sizzling inside me like a volcano. Without my knowing it was going to happen, in the middle of a session, I suddenly erupted in torrents of tears. I was embarrassed but the counsellor just smiled kindly and passed a thousand tissues.

(Keith)

- I've learned more about myself through Counselling (Organised through the Carers Association). I've come to realise I'm a 'dutiful' daughter. I didn't think I had a choice when I looked after Mum. Y'see, my father said to me: "Now if anything happens to me, you must look after your mother." So of course, whoosh, I was right in there. But I've told each of my children separately that if anything happens to me they must not feel like they have to look after their Dad. I know what a burden it is to care for him with the Alzheimer's. I wouldn't wish that on any of them. If they choose to do it, it won't be because I've said so, it won't be because of duty. It will be a choice they make because they want to do it for Dad.

(Betty, mother of four children, a carer for her mother for 11 years, now caring for husband, George, suffering from Alzheimer's)

Therapy

- I had a very good therapist. One day I said look what you've done, I feel so much better. She said, I haven't done anything. You've done it all yourself.

(Ann)

- I have been helped by Reiki, a gentle healing body-work done with your clothes on. You just lie on a table and let the Reiki do it's work.

(Michael)

Reading

Reading books about others in similar situations helped. I came to know Swraj, you are not the only man who has gone through tragedy. This helped.

(Lord Paul, father of Ambika, who died, aged four, from leukaemia)

Religion

I am religious and have found the Catholic Church to be very supportive. My faith and prayers have helped me through the hardest times. I'm in a wheelchair myself now. The church is sending me to Lourdes this summer. Also, what I find helpful, is to keep a photo of Bob by the phone. I chat away to him and tell him things. The children think I'm nuts, but it helps me.

(Maureen, a carer for her husband Bob)

Quakerism

We believe in the god within, silent worship. Prayer and meditation helped me get in touch with what I was really feeling.

(Renee)

Medical and Family Support

Caring for a severely disabled daughter, my husband and I, so close, a real team, then, suddenly, my husband died, my daughter shortly afterwards. Following these devastating losses, l became addicted to sleeping pills and passed weeks in a hazy daze and then simply stopped functioning. I needed psychiatric and specialised care. My children never gave up on me. If it were not for them, I wouldn't be alive today. My family is my strength. Two sons and a daughter who have recently admitted to me they always thought I loved Morag most of all. I didn't. They each had their own place in my heart, still do. Every one of them is special and nothing can ever replace any one of them. Some day, with children of their own, I pray they will come to recognise that I never loved any of them less because I had so much to do for the one that needed it the most.

(Helena, a carer for her daughter Morag, died age twenty-six)

Grandson

The day I held my new baby grandson in my arms was the day of my new life too. The old life had gone, the new life borne. My grandson is my source of strength.

(Margaret)

If you are grappling with grief or unresolved issues and are seeking 'something' to help you, it may be a time for experimenting, of seeing what 'fits'. Being open and willing to try things is a good start. It may be that you will try a few things before you find something that suits. Persevere. I believe this getting to know what works for us is all part of the journey. It has taken me seven years to discover the wonder of Osho meditation. A friend introduced me to it shortly after my parents died and I tried it once then soon forgot about it. It was obviously not the right time. We come to certain paths when we are ready and not before. Luckily, I discovered something else much sooner ...

Four months after my mother died, I found myself one Friday evening in a building just off Marble Arch in London. Up until then I had only had a few massages in my life. All that was about to change.

Memory — Twenty-eight years old

Enrolling in a massage course had seemed a good idea at the time. Now, in a little room with around twenty people, all ages, colours, women and men ... gosh, do we have to take our clothes off ... I mean, like, lie on the slab ... starkers? Maybe I should have checked the small print before signing the cheque?

Ted, the teacher, is waving a skeleton at us, telling us this is a metatarsal, a trapezius, a humerus, explaining that massage will release emotions, decrease toxins, increase vitality, connect mind, body, spirit and create harmony within. Ted is one of the sickliest guys I have ever seen and I can't help thinking that, of the two, the skeleton looks the healthier.

We go round the room, say our name, why we are here, what made us sign up for a massage course. Most people want to set up in business, they've heard massage is lucrative if you get into the posh hotels. Ted tells us that two of his students set up in a ski resort and made a fortune treating rich Europeans. But, he adds mysteriously, learning massage will open up a world much more than about making money. Massage will open up ourselves!

We have to get a massage buddy and I grab Karen, a dancer. She is smiley, kind-looking and is doing the massage course because she has just discovered that she has an inherited eye disease. She will go blind. She doesn't know exactly when ... her plan is, when blind, she can earn a living through touch, through massage. I am upset. Blind? How? Why? Can't they do something? Karen says no. It seems unbelievable, cruel. My own troubles momentarily forgotten and then remembered ... Karen's dilemma is yet more evidence for the shitty things that happen in this world, this miserable, torturous, unfair world.

Warm oil on bitter skin, knotted muscles, sore, soothing, oh ... shallow breath deepening, back widening, frazzled brain connecting to ... are these really my metatarsals, trapezius and ... thingummy crying out beneath your touch? Sensations humming between body brain and back again. Melting, this suit of armour, me, now surrendering, now fighting, my body, me.

"Audrey ..."

... A voice far off,

"... your turn ..."

I pretend to be asleep in the hope Karen will keep on …

"… Wakey-wakey …"

Reluctantly I open my eyes and wonder … why, oh why, didn't I discover massage long ago?

Looking back, perhaps this pull towards learning massage was with me at an earlier age. I remember once, in my teens, walking past a massage parlour and seeing a notice in the window. Staff needed. I rang the bell. A woman dressed in a mini skirt with long black hair and scarlet lip-stick unlocked the door and peered round. "I'm enquiring about the staff vacancy", I said. She said, "Do you know what we do here?" "Massage," I said. "We're fine for staff right now," she smiled and shut the door.

Oh how innocent I was!

So perhaps we have a pull towards a path, but often do not act until a major life-change triggers us to action?

If my parents had not died, I would not have been half-naked in a roomful of strangers discussing my zig-zag spine and unbalanced hips. I would have been too busy to notice.

It was amazing to look at the body in a non-sexual way. Breasts and buttocks and pelvises now became just skin and muscle, became more about what structural problems might lie beneath, how that would affect organs and the glands that governed organs, how stress and trauma sapped the life-force around the emotional centres or chakras …

Past caring I had no sense of centre. Just a cold heavy hole at my middle. Then someone touched me below the belly-button and … I wanted to curl up like a baby and cry.

I had no intentions of using massage as a way of making money. Rather I hoped I might get in touch with myself.

Despite Ted's pallid appearance, he taught wonderful massage. And Karen was the perfect buddy, her enthusiasm and zest for life (in the face of impending blindness) made learning fun. We'd go off for cappuccinos after class and test each other on the names of 'dem bones, dem bones', where, what and how they were attached. I came to discover more about myself, discover what the caffeine I gleefully threw down my neck did to my adrenals. It didn't stop me drinking it. (I had spent years fuelled by caffeine, grabbing food on the hoof.) Now, my diet was possibly worse. Toast n'banana, cheese, beans, toast n'anything, really. I couldn't be bothered to cook. Truth is, I couldn't cook. Well, not much beyond pasta and a boiled egg. Dare I say I would have learned how to cook had there not been so much illness to attend to? Or is that just a good excuse?

The fact was, at age twenty-eight, I couldn't cook and after so many years caring, it seemed much too much effort to care about me. And yet ... here I was on a massage course and now I knew what caffeine did to my poor adrenals. It didn't stop me drinking it but it was a start.

* * *

Holistic therapies, that is therapies that treat the mind, body and spirit, the whole person, are recommended at times of grief. But holistic therapies are expensive and it's not easy for carers who have lost earning potential over the years of unpaid caring.

There are some free counselling services offered for carers and past carers. There are also carers support groups all over the UK (see page 237).

With their caring days over, some people may feel they no longer wish to attend a carers support group. It is true that the needs of past carers differ from current carers. But for Ann, 66, whose son Peter died from Aids, attending the same carers support group before and after Peter died was her 'lifeline'.

Caring for someone with cancer evokes sympathy. Almost everyone at some point in life will know someone who has this disease. Caring for someone with HIV or alcoholism or drug addiction or mental illness throws up judgements.

Ann's Story

The particular support group I attended was structured around a process called co-counselling; each person has a certain amount of time to speak with absolutely no interruptions. There are no judgements, no trying to fix things, no trying to change things. Those twenty minutes where I was able to talk about how I felt *with nobody trying to make it better* played an important part in my healing. I think the thing to learn is that you can't make it better. Nobody can make it better because nobody can change what happened. Somehow by others simply being there, silently supportive, after I said my bit I did feel better.

I could say, in complete safety, thank goodness Peter is dead now. We've had eighteen years of trauma and sometimes the trauma has been horrendous and so, in a way, his death isn't really trauma. It's a relief: because it's been 'too much'. If I said that 'outside', folk might think gosh, fancy saying that, that's a weird thing to say about your son. So allowing and being allowed to be honest about where I was at without anybody judging me or trying to make it better, that's what worked for me.

I have continued with the co-counselling on a one-to-one basis, and through this, I have learned how to cry. It has taken me sixty odd years to learn to cry. I never cried when Peter died, or when my husband Jack died. Now I have learned how to access deep feelings and say oh yes, oh yes, this feels hellish and I just allow the tears to come.

It's only in the last couple of years that I have properly grieved Peter, who died in 1995.

Peter was a lovely child, but as he grew older he developed a wild, wacky side to his personality. He was difficult to handle. At the age of twelve we caught him glue-sniffing. He became addicted to solvents. This habit eventually escalated to heroin abuse in his teens.

As a mother of a heroin addict I'd often ask myself where did I go wrong that my child decided to go down that road? I have two daughters who fortunately are not into drugs. Still, I'd desperately search for a reason, to try to make sense of it. And it takes a good long while to work out that well, we all have choices. Yet even now, I'll find myself thinking oh if only *I'd* tried harder he would have kicked the habit, if only I'd tried harder ...

I say to others in similar situations look, you can't make it happen. Still, they think they can. Of course you hope, when it's someone you love you will never give up hoping that things will get better. Hope is all you have. Over and over you ask yourself what can I do, what? I knew so much anger, frustration, helplessness. Peter's habit was killing me too. I was up and down like a yo-yo. One minute I'd be trying so hard to help Peter, the next I'd be erupting like a volcano, phoning the police to come and take him out the house.

Caring for someone who is a heroin abuser is a catalogue of trauma; stealing, dealing with the police, the courts. Peter would steal something from me and sell it on to a shop. I'd have to go buy it back. He'd turn up at the school where I worked as a teacher, high as a kite hassling me to give him money. You can't hide this sort of illness neatly away, the knock-on effect seeps into all areas of your life. There were days when I'd say that's it, I'm finished with him, let him go to hell. But in the end Jack and I couldn't walk away. We couldn't jettison our son. Just couldn't do it.

When Peter was fourteen he was expelled from school. He was glue-sniffing, his behaviour erratic, he ended up in the young person's unit of the local psychiatric hospital. I didn't know where to turn. Everything got too much for me. I took an overdose and ended up in psychiatric hospital too! There was a foreign female doctor at the hospital. She said to me "Oh you Scottish women, where I come from we shout, we scream, we let it all out."

She was right. All the anger, pain, worry, I had held it all in. What comes to mind is that old-fashioned Scottish woman thing. Y'know that cultural thing, that no matter how difficult things are at home it doesn't go beyond your front door. The belief that somehow it's a weakness to ask for help so you don't, you just listen to this little voice inside that says you have to keep going, be strong, you just have to keep going and get through it. No matter what.

When I was a wee girl, crying was not allowed in my family. No matter how tough things got, it was no use feeling sorry for yourself, you just got on with it. 'Feelings' were taboo. I carried that conditioning into my adult life, choosing friends and perhaps even a husband who would not demand much from me emotionally. Jack and I loved each other but we never opened up, discussed feelings in any nitty-gritty kind of way. We just got on with whatever was happening in our lives, got on with helping Peter. There we were witnessing our son dying and we didn't – couldn't – share what it was doing to us.

Peter was twenty-four when he told me he was HIV positive. I was devastated.

I wanted to support my son but was determined to hang onto something for myself too. Jack was a headmaster, I a teacher. I enjoyed my job and was determined to keep working. Peter too, was determined to keep living in his own flat in supported accommodation and take care of himself as much as possible.

Each day after work Jack and I would go fetch Peter and take him to our house for tea. It didn't feel odd to be going to collect our adult son. Because of his addiction Peter had remained, in one way or another, ever dependent.

Christmas 1995 – I had taken Peter up-town to do his Christmas shopping. Later, at home, Peter was so weak he could barely write the wee tags for folk's presents. He knew that this was it and I knew that this was it. I wasn't in denial about him dying but again, the denial to allow myself to feel anything. I focused instead on just getting through. We didn't talk about his dying. Many of his friends had planned their own funerals, Peter and I had been to these funerals together but we did not talk about his funeral. It was just too hard. Now I would do things differently. I would broach the subject, talk to him about his leaving us, but then I couldn't. I don't beat myself up about it. I have learned to accept that was where I was at that time.

New Year came and Peter was worse. I phoned an ambulance. I don't feel guilty. It was self-preservation. I realised I didn't want him in the house. I recognised I couldn't handle it. I didn't *want* to handle it.

Our son was taken to the City Hospital where they let him go very gently. When they first started treating Aids patients there was a lot of aggressive intervention but they said they had learned more about the disease, as had all of us, over time. They had learned that by letting people go gently, it was a 'good' death. A more dignified death. Peter was in bed and we were there by his side and … it was okay. Y'know … it was okay.

At Peter's funeral we had big folding boards displaying photos of him throughout his life. We handed round cut-out paper leaves inviting people to write down how they remembered Peter. I keep the leaves in an envelope. From time to time I'll take them out and read them. Some of them are quite funny, one person had written, 'I remember all the arguments we had'.

Eight weeks after Peter died Jack fell ill. The hospital said they thought it looked like leukaemia, but then said no, it wasn't. They told him to come back in four months, so naturally we thought it couldn't be anything serious. Then, one day, quite suddenly, Jack fell severely ill. He died of septicaemia shortly after being admitted to hospital. I didn't have a chance to say goodbye. In fact, the last thing I said was, "Your toothbrush is in your toilet bag!"

Peter and now Jack, gone. I remember life was like a series of tunnels, long, dark tunnels, looming ahead with me chugging along thinking I've got to get through them, somehow I've got to get through them.

The carers' group was my lifeline. Here everyone knew what I had been through, I didn't have to explain anything. With people 'outside' I put up barriers. I avoided folk. I told myself they would find it too difficult to handle what had gone on for me, but really, I didn't give them the chance. I had to show I, Ann, was coping.

I pushed myself to go on holiday and off I went with a tour group called Solos to Croatia. I was trying to prove something to others – to myself? To say, look, I'm handling it, I'm strong, I'm away on holiday, I'm fine. 'Course I wasn't. I remember being in the group one night and one of the women got very drunk. It made me angry. I thought, I don't bloody well want to be around people who are out of their minds. I've had enough of that with Peter. I sat there, in the group, fuming. Finally one of the other women cottoned on and suggested we go for a walk.

If that happened now I would get up and leave much sooner. I would just get up and go. I would see I had a choice. But then, I just sat there feeling angry yet not doing anything to remove myself from the situation that was making me angry.

In 1999 I was diagnosed with breast cancer. There I was in a small room with two doctors and a nurse and they said, well, we've taken the tests and it's cancer. How do you feel about it? I said I am bloody angry. The nurse said that's fine, just go for it. I thought that was great. She gave me – I finally gave myself – permission to be angry. I shouted, cried, howled. All the anger I had repressed over the years surfaced – not anger about what had happened to Peter but what had happened to me, what he had put me through. Perhaps subconsciously, my body had felt it couldn't express this anger until something awful had happened to it. Well now it was time to take care of me, my body. My anger.

I went to a nutritionist and got advice. I went to a herbalist. I went to relaxation classes. I did Gestalt therapy. I had done this therapy at various times over the years and had built up quite a rapport with the therapist, a lovely lady. I devoured endless books on the subject of cancer. I was never scared I might die. Just furious at what had happened to me. I went to a cancer support group at Maggie's Centre and again, there was a real faith amongst the people there that they could both get support and be supportive, that the two are not separate but connected.

I had a mastectomy. I healed very well. I think this is because I had begun to really care for me. For so long it was a case of looking after everyone else, of just getting through. It wasn't until I got cancer that I was forced to think of myself, look after my feelings.

Accessing feelings is an on-going process. I constantly have to fight against old patterns; the habit of 'I have to get through this on my own'. I still get scared of unpleasant feelings, scared that I will disintegrate entirely, but really tears and unpleasant feelings are simply tears and unpleasant feelings. I see that now.

And in my life-journey I am learning … it is not a weakness to ask for help.

I have learned to build up pockets of support that I can dip into as required. Over the years I have from time to time used Prozac to help me keep going, although I believe medication can alleviate the symptoms it doesn't tackle the root cause. I go to the Gestalt therapy to help me work through tough times. Sometimes I'll drop into Maggie's Centre, other times I may call a member of the co-counselling group. So I am slowly learning how to take care of myself by allowing myself to be supported and cared for.

It's only in the last couple of years that I have given myself permission to grieve. That's five years of doing battle with myself, suppressing the sadness. People say time heals. I'd say not that it heals, but changes. That wound will always be there but you learn to live with, accept the wound. In accepting it there are still days when I get angry and upset. But the great thing is, because I can now access feelings, I can be angry and upset and say 'Bloody hell, I'm really angry that Peter went that way'.

I am sixty-seven now and y'know what? I'd like to have a little fun in my life. I joined a keep-fit dance class and I go to that twice a week and yes, it's fun.

When I was little I had a special dress that hung in the wardrobe and was to be kept for special occasions. That special dress was so beautiful I longed with all my heart to wear it: but no occasion special enough ever came along. My beautiful dress hung in the darkness, immaculate, unspoiled, unused until finally I had outgrown it ... I'm sixty-seven and I want to treat myself today. For no reason. No more waiting.

* * *

Recovering with Creativity

Accessing feelings can take many shapes and forms. I received the following letter:

> Dear Audrey,
> I was a full-time carer for ten years, after which my husband was in a nursing home for eight years before he sadly died last summer.
>
> I have always written poetry and short stories, just for me, my private thoughts. Not being a full-time carer any more gave me the time to type things out neatly. I decided to send them off to magazines. Amidst the rejection slips I was lucky to have a few short stories published. With the poetry, I eventually found small presses who liked my work, and one who has now published two collections.
>
> When my husband went into the nursing home I had the time to join writing groups and meet other poets. I have met some wonderful new friends through the poetry and must admit that to have my first book published when I was seventy-seven was a thrill.
> Yours,
> Elaine

Elaine shows that it is never too late to follow our dreams.

Many people use a creative form to try to make sense of a tragic event. They use it as a way of exploring what happened, to have a safe place to pour unresolved feelings. Creative work often yields insights that can give us a deeper understanding of events, of the part that we played in them. Alone, in private, or in a group, we can give ourselves space to reflect on what happened, how we felt and connect feelings of then and now.

Many past carers told me they used writing as a form of release. Writing is a wonderful way of expressing emotions, of giving them a voice, whether writing poetry, prose, a journal or even a letter. I was touched by the number of letters I received from past carers that were signed off 'I have never expressed this to anyone before and writing it down has made me feel a little better'.

Many great writers would never have written a word had a tragedy not interrupted their lives.

You don't have to be a writer to write. The important thing is to get your thoughts down, however haphazard they might be. Don't worry about 'getting it right'. There is no right – what matters is the process of writing about how we feel.

"The anger that had been building up in me added a creativity to my life and led me to writing letters to the radio and a local newspaper which gained a response."
(Margaret, from Liverpool, a carer for nine years for her father.)

Shirley, a past carer for her husband, sent me the following poem:

Words to a Carer

If you are a carer then you will know
At times you feel there is nowhere to go
From dawn to dusk you try your best
Never accepting that you need to rest.
Not always appreciated for what you do
No-one to share your point of view
Each day dawns with little hope
You just wonder if you can cope
Find someone who can understand
Keep this friend always close at hand
Talk about your doubts and fears
Don't feel ashamed of shedding tears
A carer's job is a worthwhile one
Until that sad day your caring's done.
Do not feel guilty or depressed
While you were caring you did your best,
Look back on the good times, forget the pain
And learn to live your life again!

For Renee, a creative release came in the form of music. Here, she tells how it came about …

After Bob died I went to stay with my daughter Barbara and her family for ten days. One morning Barbara said to me, "We've been invited in next door for coffee." And when we arrived at the neighbour's house, there were three very impressive keyboards all laid out. Barbara said oh look mother – keyboards! And then this woman sat down and played them absolutely beautifully. (This had all been pre-arranged, of course!) I remarked on the beauty of the music and Barbara said, "Well mother, you'd better get used to it, because we're going into Winchester tomorrow and Brian and I are buying you a keyboard!"

I am very lucky in having a close relationship with my daughter. She must have been thinking – now, what can I give mother to do? I would never have dreamed of buying a keyboard, never. And when the man in the shop demonstrated it, I thought, I'll never be able to do that. But it really did help me in the time after Bob died because it gave me something definite to work at. I bought some books to teach myself. Then, quite incredibly, I bumped into someone in the village who said, I hear you've got a keyboard. I'm learning too. How about my instructor and I come round to you and we'll learn together? It was great fun. Now, every night before bed, I play on the keyboard for Bob and me. I have discovered a talent I had no idea I had. Not only am I pleasantly surprised I can play, but it gives me much comfort too. I've played every single night since Bob died.

Other creative forms may include painting, sculpture, drama, photography. Just give it a go. Anything that allows self-expression, that frees the spirit, that channels pain in a healthy, creative way, is good.

Memory – Twenty-eight years old

It is a balmy summer's evening and I lie on the roof of the houseboat on a red blanket with a pen and small notebook in hand. I haven't written since I was a schoolchild. It feels daunting, but I need to write. What else am I to do with this 'stuff'?

The dogs, Judy, a sleek black lab and Tara, a woolly Heinz 57, snuggle on either side, happily snoozing after their long walk. Jo, the owner of the boat and the dogs, has become more friend than boat-lady and has kindly 'loaned' them to me. It makes sense. She works full-time. She is in an office whilst I am walking, walking through fields, woods, along the river towpath all the way to Hambledon and back. Some days I may be loaned a little motor boat by a neighbour who lives on the tiny island down river. This is more of an adventure as we skim speedily under Henley Bridge, the dogs on the prow like Greek statues, barking. If the weather is appalling we venture no further than the quarry opposite Ondine where rumour has it that a bunker is built into the hillside and to which the Queen will be taken in the event of a nuclear attack. It does have an eerie atmosphere and I have visions of the dogs – or myself – tumbling into a hole in the ground like Alice, except, unlike Alice, we never return.

By days I walk. I ask why. Oh God, why? I try to make sense of non-sense. In the evenings I write. I feel compelled to write poems, well, sort of poems. I know nothing about the form: nothing about rhyming or how many lines need to go where. It doesn't matter. What matters is that I spew some 'stuff' up onto the page as opposed to leaving it tangled in my intestines, festering. I don't read poetry. My reading at the moment consists of self-help books. *You Can Heal Your Life*, a present from an actress in Trainer, sits next to my bed like a Bible. There are books on bereavement, Buddhism and anything, everything to do with suffering. I am drawn to suffering. Fun, feel-good is too far-fetched. I wail buckets for the little boy Timothy Parry whose life-support machine has been switched off after being blown up by an IRA bomb. I cry at a fictional play about four women in a cancer ward. I don't cry for my parents. I go to the cinema seeking out films that have unhappy endings. Ken Loach films are great, as are French love affairs. In the dark, I relish the tragic tales. I want to leave weeping, drained. I want to feel. (I can't understand why nobody wants to go to the cinema with me.)

Henley is a place of bright young things intent on fun. Henley buzzes with parties, cocktails, balls. Nothing is taken too seriously, even death. When I told someone I had lost my parents they quipped "To lose one parent is unfortunate, to lose both is downright careless!" We laughed. I knew it to be a line from a play and the style suited the town, a place of performance and melodrama.

Looking back, although I felt alone in a sense, far from aunts, uncles, brother, sister, I was never lonely. I had chosen this place. And perhaps to be in Henley, where nothing was taken too seriously, was exactly right for me. Perhaps, in my obsession with pain and suffering and death, it was apt that I find myself surrounded by a merry throng, perhaps the tension of opposites kept me sane.

As dusk fell I would lie on the red blanket with the dogs snuggling and the swans shimmying by, and I would write poems. I would pause only to wave to the couples twisting this way and that aboard the mock Mississippi paddle steamer that would sail past every evening, a jazz band blasting. I would wave and strangers or new-found friends would wave back, shout "Join us for drinks later at the Angel?" And I would.

For, I was seeking …

"Just sex, no commitment …"

Is that me?

"No commitment, just sex …"

Me really saying that?

"… just give me sex and please leave in the morning …"

Gosh, my parents would be spinning in their graves …

WANTED – purely boudoir buddy for twenty-eight year old woman. No real boyfriend for five years. Previously two long-term relationships with faithfulness and emotional intimacy guaranteed. Sorry, not in a position to offer emotions at present. Nor am able to explain why. Will be faithful but only if you promise not to be my boyfriend.

It seemed that having been in such close proximity to death, I now had an insatiable lust for life. A longing for pure physical pleasure to make up for the deadness inside? It wasn't that I wanted to sleep with a lot of men – I didn't – I wanted one man to have sex with on a regular basis that would not involve any expectations or emotional demands of any kind. I did not want anything that remotely constituted a relationship, and I certainly didn't want a boyfriend. (My male friends joked to me later that I sounded like every man's fantasy.) The thing was, I had nothing left to give of myself emotionally. The tank was empty. Drained dry.

It just seemed a waste. I was living on a houseboat, one giant waterbed, and the summer stretched endlessly ahead. I had a bedroom whose patio windows framed the most amazing river view. There'd be a decent cup of tea (I am Scottish after all) in the morning before my bedfellow would be politely asked to leave. It may be a few days or weeks before we'd meet again.

And if it's you … when we do, don't ask me details about my life. I can't formulate sentences sometimes. My concentration is so bad I jump around when I'm talking … it's like my mind can't cope with any more thoughts, can't take in any more information. Don't ask me to make a plan for next week … it's far too far ahead. See, if someone you love is ill you can never plan anything because you don't know what's going to happen that day. You spend your life cancelling plans. So you learn to live a life of no commitment. A life of moments. I know I'm free now but it's hard to re-adjust, sorry, I just can't organise myself. Once, to act was my priority. Then, the well-being of my parents became my priority. I knew how to structure everything else in my life around that. I knew where, who, I was. Now I'm like a cell that has lost its nucleus. Don't know how to behave. There's no pecking order any more, just this huge emptiness I'm flailing around in … If I seem hyper it's just that my body is geared for emergencies. If I cry out or laugh in my sleep just ignore me … I have bad dreams … bad and funny too … like the one where I was screaming abuse at Parkinson, y'know the chat show host … in my dream my Dad was sitting there, all fat-faced and healthy again, saying, well the thing is Michael, when I agreed that you could film my dying, I really had no idea what I was letting myself in for. And I started yelling at Parkinson – he didn't know, he didn't know, you should have stopped the filming! … sometimes …

when I wake I'm not sure what's real and what's unreal … for a second I might think oh, must tell Mum that … then … by the way, it takes me all day to post a letter, so don't expect a meal.

Just come and go.

Don't expect anything.

Nothing.

I spent that summer with a guy who agreed to such an arrangement. We both went into it knowing there was an end in sight. Because there was no expectation from either side we got on better than most couples. There was no manipulation. No 'why didn't you phone me last night?' No attention-sulks. No game playing because the game was out in the open. There were no hidden agendas or using the other person for our own needs under the disguise of love. There was no treating each other badly to feel superior. There was no using sex as a weapon. There was honesty. Respect. Mutual benefit. And the day it finished we almost shook hands and said thank you.

Until my parents died I did not know that I could separate emotions from sex. I never had before. For me, the discovery was liberating. I felt empowered. Like a less-busty Madonna. A woman who made her own choices based not on society or conditioning but on what she wanted.

Past caring, my relationships with the male species fell into two distinct categories.

Men whom I thought of as good friends, who I could talk to, trust. They were caring men and I wanted to be cared for by them. They were not good for having sex with because then things would get far too complicated. I would then be in a position of having to give something back, some kind of intimate emotional care. I had nothing to give. Thus I couldn't sleep with someone who was my friend.

The second category was made up of men who were potential lovers. They were a much more selfish, self-centred species than the first. They did not want to take care of me because they were too busy taking care of themselves. They were high-achievers who had five-year plans. They appeared insensitive to emotional pain. They were not, nor could become, friends. Superficial friends yes but not real friends. So, it was safe to go to bed with them.

Oh how I longed to be cared for – and yet remain carefree.

I couldn't imagine ever being close, able to give emotionally to anyone ever again. If there is no love in your own heart how can you give it? If you are empty inside how can you fill someone else up?

You can pretend to. But I was finished with pretending. The only way I might have somebody in my life and make it work was to be brutally honest about my lack of feeling.

And so, that summer, the first past caring, I embarked on a brief encounter. And although it didn't take the pain away – what could? – I looked forward to those late-night visits.

But first I would write on the roof, on the red blanket, tea-cups scattered like stepping stones, I would write

A POEM, sort of

I read once in a play the final words the actress spoke,
"I've always relied on the kindness of strangers," she said.
I didn't quite understand it, thought it was a joke.

But now I see it clearer, with insight full and deep,
As friends fulfilled their world, mine crumbled, decayed.
I prayed. No-one heard, God, even, asleep.

Friends far away, too busy with work/to talk/abroad
So I turned to new faces, eager to help, please
And I felt eased.

And I talked with folks I only knew because they lived so
Close, up-river, across bridges. Strange strangers listened
As I poured out more, more: tales of woe.

And I told these new-found faces huge chapters of my tale,
Yet hardly talked to friends at all. Strangers all
Listened gravely over dinner/drinks/nibbles, mostly male.

And friends were busy, too busy to pay a visit/write/phone
But it mattered not for I was not alone.
Geographically sow the seeds and instant friends are grown.
Yet how can these people truly be called friends?
They know nothing of me but that I live nearby.
And I speak of a heart torn: a heart that never mends.

Still, strangers come and offer an ear/a meal/a bed
But where are my friends, my history, why don't they come?
My schedule is too busy is what the voices said.

And so I turn to strangers because they live close by,
They see the tip of iceberg years. They never see me cry.
I turn to the stranger in myself: core hardened, harder, try …

Try to shrug, tell the world to fuck off
I'll survive, keep my story buried deep inside
But talking to strangers I get soft, soft.

But talking to strangers gets me nowhere.
They don't know me, me of time shared/fears/cared
So how can they understand and is it really fair?

I don't care.
Yet other times I do. Feel abandoned/in despair
Perhaps friendships build barriers that are by strangers –
    broken –
Because strangers walk away/move on/come, go – often.

"I've always relied on the comfort of strangers," the actress
said,
As she pulled back the covers and got into bed.

* * *

Several years ago I was having a coffee with a friend of mine, Gabriel. I told him I was writing a book. "Oh yeah?" he grinned. "Lots of sex, drugs n' rock n' roll, I hope."

"Er ... not exactly ... it's about caring," I replied.

"Oh," was all he said, before we talked of other things.

Four months later, he called to tell me his lovely wife Susie had been diagnosed with a rare form of cancer. Gabriel cared for her. Tragically, she died within ten months of the diagnosis.

After Susie died, Gabriel enquired how the book was going. "I've not been doing much work on it," I admitted.

"You've got to write it," he insisted. "Listen, I want to tell you something. When you told me you were working on a book about caring, I thought, how boring, that'll never sell, what's Audrey bothering with that for? But now, having been through it, it's got to be written, so get on with it."

(Gabriel knows I love to procrastinate!)

Unfortunately, it's not until something happens to us, that we can truly understand it.

"Don't judge someone until you've walked at least a mile in their shoes," Atticus tells his children in Harper Lee's classic book *To Kill A Mockingbird*.

Unfortunately we live in a society where we judge and are judged every single day on our 'external selves'. On job status, size of house, car, wallet, on what we wear, on how we look. We live in a world where we are judged by what we do, rather than who we are *being* in life. A world where sadly the work of carers goes unrecognised.

Every past carer I spoke to told me they experienced severe loss of self-esteem.

Mary told me: "I would walk down the street and I felt I couldn't hold my head up. I felt so worthless. Everyone else had something to show for their life. I felt I had nothing to show."

Loss of confidence is scary. When we feel insecure or inadequate the instinct is to spend all our time either fighting or defending. It is difficult, especially in our competitive world, to allow ourselves to simply sit with our feelings of vulnerability.

Loss of confidence, if explored in a healthy way, can often give us new insights about ourselves. I would never have done this book had I not suffered such a drastic loss of confidence. I chose writing as a way of channelling my pain. I was bitter and confused and angry and sad and I didn't know what else to do so I wrote and wrote and wrote and I felt better. The purpose of my writing was served by the very act of writing. It was sore, raw and a balm to my bloody wounds. It hurt like hell and gave relief. It shook me up and freed me up.

Our pain is ours, so why be afraid of it? Get to know your pain, invite it in. Only by allowing ourselves – giving ourselves permission to feel our pain completely – may we be able to pass through it, catch a glimpse of what lies beyond. When we explore our pain, we discover things about ourselves. I discovered writing.

*   *   *

I asked a group of past carers what they had discovered about themselves:

- I now listen to people, really listen, I never did before. When I first moved here, in an attempt to get to know some of my neighbours, I'd pop in for the odd cup of tea. I became quite friendly with a lady across the road – she had lost her husband some years before. When I visited she would talk incessantly about her husband, for hours and hours. This went on for three years. Then, gradually, she began to talk of other things. I didn't mind sitting there, because I realised that probably no one had ever listened to her before. I suppose my experience of caring for Mum has made me more compassionate, more willing to listen, more prepared to give up my time for another. Now this lady has really moved on and has joined CRUSE. So she is helping others now to come to terms with bereavement.

(Betty)

- I am a more generous person than I was before. I no longer hold grudges or entertain petty squabbles. Caring has made me more aware of death. Life's too short for not speaking.

(Eleanor)

- Before I had an opinion about "carers" as being little old ladies and men, now I am one myself I see carers are people like you and me. Just people, really.

(Gabriel)

- Time is precious to me now. I know death and illness can come any day, so I no longer want to waste it.

(Eric)

- I would never have taken up teaching if I hadn't had a handicapped daughter.

(Mildred)

- I feel more for others now. I am more caring in every sense.

(Keith)

- Friendship and people are more important to me now than work. At the end of the day, we need each other more than we need money.

(Margaret)

- I was a man used to being in control of my life. Now I was out of control. In caring I had to learn how to be vulnerable.

(Lewis)

When I contacted Lewis to ask if he would be willing to be interviewed, he suggested straight away that we should meet and that he would take me to lunch. I pointed out that although a very kind invite, as the author, I really ought to be treating him to lunch. He wouldn't hear of it. I forgot that I was talking to a seventy-five year old Scotsman for whom the idea of a lady paying for her own lunch, or even more unthinkable, paying for a gentleman's, did not rest easy.

Yet for Lewis, who spent his working life in the high-powered corporate world as Director of Finance at Scottish Television (he was later awarded an OBE), the news of his wife Greta's diagnosis with Alzheimer's brought a role-reversal. For not only did Lewis care for Greta but also took care of the cooking, cleaning and shopping in the way that Greta once had.

Meeting Lewis reminded me of my own father. How he, together with my brother, had devotedly taken care of Mum and the home. How frustrated my mother had been. These chores, she considered, were her domain.

Nowadays, there is perhaps a sense of bewilderment in how any woman can be satisfied "just looking after a man, home and children" but for my mother, I know, her modest bungalow and we, her children, were a constant source of pride.

Now it is expected men will know how to cook and clean. If both partners are healthy, domestic chores are usually shared. This is the generation I grew up in. It is easy to forget that in men like Lewis and my father's day, the man was the breadwinner not the breadmaker.

Over lunch, as Lewis spoke of applying make-up to Greta, I had a vivid image of my father putting lipstick on my mother, her favourite bright red lipstick that smelt of roses. How my mother would not be able to keep her lips straight for laughing and how my father would affectionately scold her, keep still, keep still, how he would dab gently with a white tissue where her mouth hung limp and the red had bled and how sometimes, only sometimes, my mother's laughter would then suddenly turn to tears.

I had this image, and others. My father shopping in Safeways, eagle-eyed, comparing bargains. My father hanging out the washing, my mother eagle-eyed, peering through the patio window to make sure the pegs were positioned just-so to catch the optimum breeze.

As I spoke to Lewis, I realised that I had not really appreciated how my father was a man of a different generation and that cooking, cleaning, running a home, were not taught to men as they are now. I had been so consumed in my own grief and confusion concerning Mum's strokes that I simply did not have the capacity to stop for a moment and imagine what the impact of her illness must be like for my Dad. One minute his beautiful wife right as rain, the next speechless, paralysed. I didn't stop to ask how he was coping. I was blind to see what a great job he was doing.

How I wished my Dad could have been sitting there at lunch so that I may have told him Dad, I think the way you cared for Mum and us, was tremendous. I'm so proud of you.

As Lewis spoke of cleaning, I had visions of my flat. My flat, as any of my friends will vouch, is in a state of continual chaos. I am averse to washing dishes. I will pay someone to hoover. There is no food in my cupboard. It's not unusual for me to turn up at various aunts' houses, around tea-time, requesting, like a beggar, a plate of hot broth. If only I had been more appreciative of what skills my mother – and latterly my father – were able to pass on to me, and not taken it, them, so much for granted, I may by now be able to make my own plate of broth. But then: Perhaps, deep down, there is a part of me that wants to remain like a hungry pup trotting off to anyone who will feed her, who will give her a soft cushion to sleep on and take good care of her. Just like home sweet home.

Like a light coming on, now I see. How I resisted – felt incapable? –of creating a home of my own after my parents died. Instead, I carted umpteen bin-bags between one set of friends to the next, staying with them for weeks, months, becoming part of the family, dipping in and out of their lives and dramas as if some extra on the set of *The Waltons*. "Here comes the bag lady," my friends would cry and in I'd trail longing to belong, looking to be cared for. And I may have moaned about all this trundling around, but like a true bag lady, didn't I also enjoy the fact that I was free of responsibilities?

So it was, in talking to other carers, I came to learn more about myself.

Lewis told me what he had learned about himself caring and past caring.

Lewis's Story

Caring instilled in me an incredible sense of humility. I was never arrogant, but I did have certain goals and ambitions that drove me to succeed in the business world. I demanded impeccable standards from both others and myself. I liked order, structure, work tasks to be completed on time. I'd get very impatient when things didn't go according to plan.

Greta's illness put all that into perspective. You can yield no control over illness.

I was capable of cleaning the house and cooking (after a few careful lessons!) and choosing nice outfits for Greta to wear, and became quite a dab hand with the make-up brushes, but I had no say in the way the disease took hold of my beloved Greta. It doesn't matter how powerful, how glamorous, how much money you have in the bank, illness makes us realise how vulnerable and helpless we really are.

From being someone who had organised my life around meetings and appointments, sometimes planned weeks, months ahead, I had to learn the humble act of acceptance. Accepting that I could not control life, could not control how my lovely wife was going to feel that day, or how much more of 'my Greta' the terrible illness may have stolen away. I had to learn to live day to day, totally in the present, dealing with the unknown as it came up. It's ironic that, with the process of dying we have no choice but to let go and trust in the process of life.

I know it sounds a cliché but illness really does remind us how fragile life is. My experience of caring taught me to take nothing and no one for granted.

I was a wee bit guilty of falling into that old trap we can so easily do with loved ones – we just assume they'll be around forever. Sometimes we only half-listen to them, one eye fixed on the television or the newspaper. Faced with the dreaded prospect of losing Greta made me painfully aware of just how precious she was to me. The simplest things, like going for a walk together, suddenly took on a whole new meaning.

I've tried to hold onto that sense of appreciation in my life after Greta's death, in that I now make a conscious effort not to take anyone for granted, whether it be my children, friends, neighbours or strangers I encounter in everyday life. And where possible I let them know they are appreciated. I simply tell them. Often it's not until someone is dying that we are reminded just how much we truly love them and how important it is to tell them so. Now I don't wait for them to be dying!

After Greta died I couldn't bear to see anyone. I'd get up with the lark and race to the supermarket, praying I wouldn't bump into anyone. If I saw lots of couples out and about I'd get terribly upset – it highlighted the pain of losing Greta. I stopped going to M&S on a Friday because it was full of couples! Silly I know, but that's what I did. I'd get in the car and drive around for hours, get out at some remote spot and go for a walk.

Good friends would call and invite me out but I'd make up some excuse or other. Several knock backs down the line, the invitation would be issued as a gentle command: "We're coming to get you, be ready at six." I would be. And to my surprise I would end up enjoying myself.

After years of feeling quite isolated as a carer it is daunting to have a 'social' life again. It can feel quite overwhelming. I am eternally grateful to those special friends who wouldn't take no for an answer and who kept coming back to me (in the face of apparent rejection), with gentle love and support. Now I'm stronger I try to show the same kind of dedication to others who are in similar circumstances, maintaining contact with them throughout, no matter what. And in my capacity as chairman of Crossroads, if I get a call saying that someone needs to talk, I'll go immediately. Before I would have thought, oh, I'll go in a few days. Now I go now.

Caring for someone who is ill can be quite a test of friendship. One friend took to coming every Tuesday for the five years that Greta was ill. Every week he would let himself in and watch telly if I was busy with Greta. He never told anyone that he came. I don't even think his wife knew. But he was there, sure as clockwork, sitting in my lounge, every Tuesday. Never a truer saying, a friend in need...

But some friends did drift away shortly after Greta's illness was diagnosed. One couple in particular, whom we had been quite close to, lost touch with us altogether, despite my efforts to keep contact. Shortly after Greta's death, a four-page letter from them fell through my door. A letter full of pain and guilt, expressing their regret at severing contact, but explaining how they simply could not deal with Greta's deteriorating condition. It frightened them. Being around illness and death can be scary and so, along with many others, they had run from it. But their guilt in doing so was catastrophic.

I knew immediately what I had to do. I picked up the phone. They were surprised to hear from me, thinking I would bear a grudge, but I didn't. I know, too, that Greta would not want it that way.

You cannot force illness on other people. Some cope better than others. If you are caring for someone you love you often find the strength and courage from a place deep inside. But, as I explained to my friends who had suffered five long years, torturing themselves over their loss of contact with us, if only they had picked up the phone and voiced their fears. If only they had made a simple five minute call to say "We're thinking about you, we just find it hard to be with you," we would have understood and not felt so completely cut off without reason. There was a lesson there that we all learned – that when we feel afraid of illness and death not to be afraid to voice it, to communicate with each other.

Shortly afterwards, when a mutual friend (who had been a regular visitor of Greta's) fell ill with stomach cancer, the wife of this couple went to visit her every day till the day she died.

The turning point in feeling better happened quite accidentally. I remember … it was just over a year since Greta died. There was an art exhibition showing locally and I'd walked past many times, thinking about going in but never quite getting there.

This particular afternoon though, I went in. I browsed 'round the paintings and was just leaving when I saw a lady I knew from my local Church. She was also on her own. She said she was going on to see another exhibition further up the hill and why not come along? I did.

Afterwards, over a cuppa in the gallery café (somewhere I would never have gone if I'd been on my own), she remarked to me, "I'm so glad I met you. What a difference it made going round with somebody, being able to chat about the paintings."

I felt like I'd turned a corner. For the first time in ages I'd had a pleasant afternoon and I felt the better for it. Also, knowing that I'd given somebody else some support, companionship, felt good too. When I told my daughter, she said "Okay Dad, now there's your answer. Stop saying no to invitations and go with it." Now my friends are surprised at how readily I accept invitations, without the usual need to be coaxed.

I think the secret is not waiting for others to take the initiative, but to reach out to one another. To realise that we are not islands, but a community. It's a shame our society seems to have lost the sense of community that it once had. Once, you knew you'd be welcome to just drop in to your neighbour's house for a quick chat over a cup of tea. Now it seems everybody is so busy these days, you need an appointment.

Y'know what I think a good motto to life is? If you can, just do it. So much time is spent procrastinating but we never know what's around the next corner, so don't put off until tomorrow what you can do today.

My beloved Greta and I were married forty-seven years. When the doctors told us of Greta's illness, I was devastated but also relieved that we had been lucky enough to do so many wonderful things together.

Y'see, shortly after I had retired we decided to splash out and treat ourselves to a three-month world trip. There is no way that we could have possibly undertaken something like that at the time of Greta's diagnosis. It would have haunted me forever to look back and think, 'I wish we'd done …' or 'if only'. Often fears stop us humans from fulfilling our potential. If there is one thing I have learned it is that disease is merciless. It doesn't give you the chance to replay lost opportunities.

> So, if you can...
> ...today
>
> *Just do it!*

Memory – Thirty years old

It's the images that haunt me. The sight of my Uncle James flapping a tartan dishcloth in front of my mother's face in a vain attempt to make air, that she may breathe. My father, in intensive care, his eyes dazed then wild, as he realised where he was. Trying to pull out the green tube in his throat, his mouth strapped open like a form of torture. Unable to speak his wishes. It's the images, those and others, of my parents' suffering that play over and over in my mind, a vivid film that plagues my every waking hour, refusing to be switched off. It's the memories that drain me. Crush me. They don't fade.

I sit on a verandah surrounded by palm trees, a stray black cat meows indignant at my feet. The sun warms me, warms my pale skin, paler still from the long dreich Scottish winter. I am plastered meticulously from head to foot in Factor 25 sunblock, organic (no harmful chemicals). I pat the bundle of fur now rubbing merrily back and forth against my bare legs - then panic: what if it's 'got something?' I notice a tiny indication of a weepy eye and instantly withdraw my hand. I adjust my baseball cap, pulling it down over my face to offer maximum protection, fix my dark sunglasses (100% UV protection guaranteed) and gaze out over the silvery blue that is the Mediterranean. A cool breeze blows from the North African coast. I close my eyes. I wonder, was I always like this? Always so scared, so fearful. I have come on holiday to relax and now I'm more worried than ever about catching skin cancer or rabies or the plane crashing or whatever.

The pleasant numbness that I had basked in, been protected by for the first year or so past caring, had given way to fear. Fear of life. Death. Of getting ill. Fear of what happened to my parents happening to me. Or indeed anyone.

This fear sapped my life-force. I would rush to the doctor at the slightest blemish, convinced I was dying. I prayed on airplanes that went through turbulence, convinced any minute we'd be crashing into the sea. It was as if I was waiting … waiting for something awful, deathly, to happen. This anxiety was exhausting. Forever feeling sick, mind reeling. Regrets... I never owned a house to invite my parents to, nor a child for them to hold, hardly had anything to show them for my life, too late now, too late. At night in bed, body sinking as if into a swamp... Struggling to breathe. My friends call me intense, say that I have lost my sense of humour, that they have never seen such a worrier. I worry about that.

I had come out of retreat and moved back to London. I had thought okay, now get a life, Audrey. I was back in the city I knew so well, the city where I had once thrived on the buzz, but now it was stressful. I was terrified when the tube broke down and we were stuck in a tunnel, sardine-like, airless. What was happening? A bomb? An accident? Any minute now a train might collide into us from behind! I was scared walking down the street. I felt incomplete, like an apple that had been de-cored.

I got offered a job again acting. Oh what a horrible experience! I didn't know what to do with the character, didn't trust myself to make a decision, had lost all sense of judgement. Worse, of instinct. I was hopeless in the part. My confidence now completely shattered. My fears were confirmed – I couldn't act anymore.

"What do you do?" people would ask.

"Nothing," I would reply. Once I was proud of that. Now I knew only a deep sense of failure.

Everybody had said it takes two years. Grief. Then you'll begin to feel better.

What idiot had come up with the two-year figure? With each day that went by I missed my parents more, not less.

I was living in a basement flat-share with three Aussie couples who had obviously decided that renting out the extra large cupboard would be a great way to supplement their weekend flights to 'do Europe'. The room was dark, dingy and had prison bars on the frosted window. It would have been more apt for a mushroom, but, still searching for 'meaning', I perhaps took the room as a way of saying, look, I have no need for materialistic comfort. See how we spend our lives on these things and yet they have no meaning.

(I have learned … A little luxury is the icing on the cake. Delicious!)

I was dating a man at that time I had met on a train. He was American, working as a management consultant, who flew all over Europe. (Ah … as I write, I see it is almost the same script as before. How easy it is to repeat ourselves.) We would meet for roughly one weekend out of three either in London or abroad. This was perfect, for the dating 'arrangement' that had come into being after my parents died seemed to have become stuck in my throat like a broken record. It became a pattern, a safety-net, a catch-phrase. 'Don't get close, don't plan, nothing to give, nothing lasts, just live for today.'

It was odd to be dating someone so successful - and someone who cared about being seen to be successful - whilst I was in the thick of my nihilistic period. Angry, lost, I wanted to wipe smiles off shiny faces.

When my American man told me about his performance bonus or a new contract his company had won, I would shake my head and start talking about starving children in Africa, orphanages in the Ukraine. When he invited me to join him on his work treat (all expenses paid yachting cruise around the South of France) I would tell him no, I couldn't possibly go, I was much too busy to be wasting time in the south of France. Then I would retreat to my miserable little room and bury myself in self-help books that told me yes, yes, – good can come from suffering.

I could not see how any good could come out of such suffering as my parents endured. I thought, people have to make up this kind of thing. They have to say that good comes of suffering. Otherwise life would be unbearable. Still, I devoured such books. I was desperate. I needed to believe it.

Meanwhile my American man and I continued in some kind of power game.

He loved designer clothes; I deliberately 'dressed-down'. He liked fine wines, I bought Tesco plonk. He was concerned with being seen in Soho's cool bars, I preferred a greasy spoon caff. What was I doing? Trying to change him. To say look, can't you see all this is worthless?

Looking back, what a royal pain in the ass I was. A self-righteous, judgmental little Missy who, because she felt such a failure, had to spoil the fun for others. The truth was, I felt so low, so inadequate that it would have been cringeworthy to be around a bunch of bright young things in France. For as much as I was rejecting society, as much as I thought I was above it all, I wasn't. It was one thing to decide not to ride on the merry-go-round, quite another to want to but not be able to climb on. I felt isolated, alone, no longer part of life, desperate to find some kind of identity that when people asked what I did, I could say "I'm a eh …"

"Get married," said a friend, "then you're a wife."

"Have a baby," said another, "you're a mother."

Yet I had no interest in either. As my friends apparently rejoiced in settling down, running homes, raising children, the things that for many people give them a sense of meaning, of purpose, I flapped my wings harder, vowing past caring nothing would clip them again.

Caring for children and caring for the dying have similar demands. There are sleepless nights with cries in the dark for you to go running … NOW! There are days passed in a blur, zombie-like, snappy, irritated, no time to go to the toilet, busy doing for someone else. I trusted my worn out bleary-eyed friends who said it was all worth it for the first word, the goofy smile, the little life that would need something from them for the next twenty years or more. I sometimes wondered if they had had children for no other reason than to fill the void in their own life, to experience the need to be needed. Past caring, I had no need of that. I doubted whether I ever would again.

But then … what did I have need of? What could break this paralysis? If I don't want to settle down, have no pull toward marriage, children, and if I have lost faith in what once was my career, worse, faith in myself, what happens next?

"How are you?"

"Fine."

My brother would call. My sister would call. I would call them. We rarely talked of our parents. It was too painful to talk of them.

"What have you been doing?" My brother would ask.

"Oh lots," I'd say.

"What have you been doing?" I'd ask my brother

"Oh … this and that."

My brother had been running his own business when my mother died. Whilst I had stopped and gone into retreat, he had kept going, working long hours to hold everything together. He had since sold his business and now had *time*. I suspected he was now going through his own period of burnout. My sister had a young family. She had had to keep going but it didn't mean that the effects of grief were not taking their toll emotionally. Still, when we called each other, we were all 'fine'. Until one day, late at night on the phone to my brother, my resolve broke.

"I miss them so much … I … don't know what to do …"

"Well come home. Just come home," my brother was saying.

"I'm fine," I blubbed.

I didn't want to go home. Two people were missing at home.

"I just want you to know I'm here for you," my brother was saying.

"I'm here for you too," I squeaked, too cheery.

"Don't worry about me."

"How's Fiona?"

"Fine."

"I'm worried about her," I told my brother.

"I'm worried about you," he told me.

"But are you really okay?" I asked him.

"Fine. You?"

"Fine."

That's how it was. Broken children trying to play parent.

"So …" my brother asked again. – "What have you been up to?"

I didn't know. Days slipped away. I seemed busy but doing … what?

Oh yes, one day a week I went to see a student counsellor. My GP had organised it, I didn't think I needed counselling(!) but went because it gave me somewhere to go. Also, I had a need to tell my story over and over. Pity the casual strangers I met on buses, trains, planes. On holiday? Yes. My parents are dead. They were both ill y'see and we were up, up and I was away.

"Do you feel angry with your parents?" the counsellor, a Greek student with charcoal hair would ask in a hushed hypnotic voice.

"No."

"Really?"

"… Well … I wish Mum hadn't smoked. I wish Dad had gone for his check-ups … but I mean, non-smokers die and people who go for their check-ups die. I'm angry they suffered so much."

"You're not angry with them?"

I sure as hell was angry at the world. Was I angry at the world because I was subconsciously angry with my parents?

One sunny afternoon, sipping coffee in Belsize Park, I was speaking of my Mum's stroke and the work we did as a family to try to help her speak again and my Californian management consultant put his hand on my leg and said,

"Well, well, aren't you the little martyr? When my grandmother became ill and in need of care, my father put her in a home."

"Why didn't your parents look after her?" I asked, shocked.

"Because they had four young children. They didn't think it would have been fair to us. They didn't want her being ill to ruin our lives."

He said – "Didn't you think of putting your mother in a home?"

I laughed – "You never met my Mum! You think you could have put her in a home?"

I laughed but it suddenly occurred to me that it had never occurred to me. Never occurred to any of us, her children. It may seem rather naive, but the thought never entered our minds. I don't necessarily think there is anything wrong with choosing to put someone who is ill and in need of care in a home (so often it depends on personalities and circumstances) yet it was so much not an option that it never existed as an option for us.

It occurred to me that putting my mother in a home would have solved nothing. It would have solved nothing because I would have wanted to be at the home day and night. I wanted to be there if my parents were ill, not because of any moral duty but simply because to be elsewhere felt wrong. If I had been acting and Mum in a home, life itself would have felt wrong. In that moment I saw I had done not what was right by my parents, but rather what was right by me. And my loss was huge. Two great people. Forever irreplaceable. What they went through forever unchangeable. And I felt not anger, but overwhelming sadness. For them and me. So much bloody sadness.

"You need a job," my brother said

"Doing what?" I said

"Anything."

I would retreat to my dungeon armed with newspapers. I would browse through the job sections and with each bizarre job title my fear would grow. What the hell was a Digital Preservation Officer, a Flash Designer, a Patent Translator? How could I get a job when I didn't even understand the job titles? It was scary 'out there'. Best to hide in my wee dark room and read my books and wait patiently until the next weekend where I could live a bit through someone else.

* * *

Work

Finding a job again after many years caring can bring up tremendous fear.

When we are doing a job we love, receiving praise and recognition from colleagues, our confidence increases. This feeling of feeling good about ourselves, of earning money for our time, our skills, feeds into our sense of who we are. If we feel good about what we do and are validated by others, we often seek to develop our skills further.

The skills carers hone over the years often go unnoticed when they are stuck within four walls. They may rarely hear anyone tell them, well done, you are doing a great job. No wonder then self-confidence suffers a severe blow.

When past carers attempt to re-enter the world of mainstream employment they are often met with prejudice. With a glaring gap in the CV, many carers never get to the interview stage. Of those who do, some wish they never had.

Mary's Story

Mary, an amazing lady from Wales, cared for a mind-blowing thirty years. Mary cared from the age of twenty-one to fifty-one, through her twenties, thirties, forties, those years where we may marry, divorce, give birth, take on a mortgage, pay into a pension, forge career, change career, where we often live to work, earn money, promotion, status, then, perhaps, work to live, to value money less and time with our loved ones more.

Mary had not been able to earn a penny in thirty years and had no savings, stocks, pension fund or nest-egg to look forward to. She desperately needed work. She applied for countless jobs. But with each rare interview came a letter of rejection.

> One interviewer asked me how would I manage to get up in the morning to come to work when I had 'not worked' for so long? And at yet another interview I was questioned as to how would I accept discipline in the work-force from supervisors, how would I be able to cope with this after being 'my own person' for so long?
>
> I began to feel it was impossible to convince prospective employers that I was a suitable person for work. In my experience prospective employers don't seem to perceive past carers as having much to offer in the traditional workplace. Don't perceive us as having loads of patience, stamina, understanding, ability to work under pressure, motivated when exhausted, conscientious and caring about our 'work' round the clock. We can't phone in a sickie when we want a day off. Carers can keep working under less than perfect conditions and require flexibility to fulfil the particular demands of each day. Carers have to remain calm in times of great stress, and are called upon to make instant decisions knowing it may be a matter of life or death …
>
> I should have thought they were all good qualities in any workplace.

To continue caring professionally is honourable if truly a choice. I was outraged, however, to hear how many past carers were pushed by well-meaning friends, advisors, carers' organisations even, into yet more caring because 'that's what you're good at'. Past carers ought to be encouraged to say okay, I may be good at it, but is it good for me? Does it suit me to continue caring? Or is there something else I wish to explore for my life now?

Many carers need a gentle nudge to remember deep, long-forgotten dreams. Support at this time is crucial. With the loss of confidence that comes with long-term caring, many people feel that they have nothing to offer apart from their caring. A view, sadly, that is too often reinforced by others.

Mary explains:

> I mentioned to a neighbour I was having difficulties in finding work and she replied, 'Well you don't expect to find work easily do you? What have you got to offer anyone?' Her words were like a knife in me. I thought Oh God, is that how other people see me? I felt so belittled, so no-good.

This chance remark was a life-changing moment for Mary. She vowed to prove to the world – to herself – that she was capable of doing other things with her life. After thirty years of caring, at the age of fifty-one, Mary embarked on what she calls her 'journey of self-actualisation'.

Disillusioned but not beaten by the negative responses from prospective employers, she applied to university to study a BSc Econ degree in Health and Social Care. In her fifties, Mary became a full-time student. She successfully attained the degree. She gained a diploma in Clinical and Pastoral Counselling. She did a postgraduate certificate in Education and Training.

Mary wrote to me, in July 1998:

> 'Even after attaining the degree I am back on income support. I still do not have paid employment. I will not give up. I hope, one day, to teach counselling skills or adults with learning difficulties.'

In autumn 2002, I travelled to meet Mary in her South Wales hometown.

As we climbed the steep hill to one of the many colleges where Mary now teaches, she reeled off her weekly schedule, making me feel doubly giddy: Mondays it's teaching young men with special needs living skills and confidence building; Tuesdays it's teaching computer skills to parents of children with disabilities; Wednesdays it's teaching counselling on the Diploma in Welfare Studies; afternoons it's back to computer skills; evenings it's off to teach the Advanced Counselling module; Friday it's computers then on to teach the Open College Network Counselling course. Saturday mornings it's counselling couples and families at Cross Keys. Sunday it's catching up with her studies with Home Fellowship Wales Distance Learning and Christian Ministry. She is currently doing a doctorate in Metaphysics.

Phew! … and she still finds the time to enjoy a loving, caring relationship with Tony, her first 'proper' boyfriend.

I had no sooner returned home and a card popped through my letterbox: Audrey, since our get-together, I now teach on the Access to Nursing Course and the Diploma in Caring. This is for young people training to work in residential care for the elderly and children. So all these caring years are now an asset because knowledge is passed on to others working in a caring environment."

For a lady who supposedly had nothing to offer, Mary has surmounted her own expectations. "I can't believe it," she tells me, giggling. "I sometimes have to pinch myself to see that it's real. I thoroughly enjoy my job, my life. It's great to be happy."

Not that Mary has regrets about caring. "To see a smile was a wonderful thing when someone was so ill and could no longer communicate. It was a hard life, but a rewarding one."

Eleven years past caring, at the age of sixty-two, Mary is revving up as others slow down, relishing that her work is still dedicated to improving the quality of life for others. "When I teach computers, I think perhaps this will provide a gateway for this person to get a job. When I teach counselling I think of this person going out into the world to help others. When I teach young men with special needs, I remind them they have a voice, an opinion, that is as valid as anyone's. I'm a teacher. I share my knowledge and my skills with others and the hope is that they will move on and do the same."

Mary teaches not merely from textbooks, but experience. She has stood right there, on the tracks. This gives her courage. The courage to speak out. She tells me:

> I found the attitude of some students very difficult to accept when I brought up Carer issues during class discussion on welfare law. It seemed many students planning to work in health or social care had no concept of what it was like to be a long-term carer, the stress involved. The attitude was that the carer had made the choice to care so they should not complain. I pointed out that sometimes the carer does not really have a choice, especially those caring from a young age. Some said 'try having a couple of kids, then you'd know what stress is'. Even some staff said that if I wanted to belong to the 'real world' I'd better toughen up. It makes me think this is why health and social care services can sometimes fail users of services. In some of the training, the perception of 'carers', the trials they face lacks real empathy. Real understanding.

Fuelled only by her faith, Mary refused to give up or shut up. Instead she spoke of her own experiences as a carer, of how certain laws may work on paper, but not in practice. She spoke up, even when laughed at, ridiculed. "I would take the sad and ignorant remarks made by others and scrape them off afterwards," she says.

Her tenacity paid off when, during teacher training, she was invited to give a lecture to a roomful of healthcare professionals.

> I stood up at the front of the room and was able to highlight two major issues that had been a bone of contention for me as a carer. There is a supposed confidentiality rule yet I often overheard nurses gossiping about other patients. I was able to say "Look, confidentiality ought to mean just that."
> The second thing was the nurses would say to me, "Oh Mary when your caring days are over you'll have to come with us for a night out. We'll take you to see a show, go for a drink." Carers cling to that, it is a hope, a plan for the future, you will be going somewhere with someone. But the day of the death,

the nurses, doctors, the home carers, all the people who have become more like friends, pull out. Move on to the next patient. Yet who cares for the carer? Nobody asked me how I would manage financially, emotionally, cognitively. Words, promises are easily forgotten. The phone remains silent. I learned people sometimes say things just to make conversation. But carers cling to this. So if you don't mean it, don't say it, I could say. It felt good to be up there at the front of the room like maybe I'd made a difference for someone else.

Mary tells her story here in the hope of making a difference. It is for all the people who hurt behind closed doors, who deserve to be told what a great job they did or are doing and who, most of all, may need to be reminded of just how much they have to offer the world.

Something about Mary: an interview

How did you come to be caring for your parents, Mary?

Until age eight, I was a happy child, carefree. Then come the memories … my mother, unwell, my grandmother, who lived around the corner coming to look after her and me. Age eleven, and suddenly my grandmother died. I learned to cook, clean, wash and iron clothes, do the shopping, look after my mother. Mother suffered from heart problems and the brittle bone disease osteoporosis. She spent long periods of time in hospital. She would later go on to develop, in her fifties, the dreaded disease Alzheimer's. My father was an engine driver for the Great Western Railway, he worked shifts and nights. I missed school. The welfare services came. They said I should go to a Children's Home in Hayling Island. They said I was in need of care myself. I kicked up a fuss, refused to leave my beloved parents. Lucky I am stubborn. I stayed home.

Officially, I left school age fifteen. I went to work in a draper's shop but my real dream was to become a nurse. I delayed applying for nurse training due to my mother's health. Twenty years old and I could delay it no longer. I felt life's chances were passing me by! I applied, was accepted and excitedly left home to pursue my career specialising in burns and orthopaedic nursing.

My father went through a red signal at Didcot station. There was an official inquiry. My father said he had had divided concentration that day because he had left a sick wife at home. Half his mind was on the job, the other on his wife. He said his only daughter had left home to become a nurse. He had no other support.

Walking down the ward carrying a bedpan, feeling guilty, so guilty, thinking I am here caring for strangers when really I am needed at home. I decided to give up my nursing training temporarily and return home to care for my mother until my father retired. He would then become the full-time carer and I would return to complete my training. I should only be home for a matter of months. I sadly bade farewell to my nursing friends. Matron reassured me there would always be a job for me. But … out the blue, shortly after I returned home, my father suffered a massive coronary. Now two sick people to care for! There appeared no way out. Only death seemed a way out. Theirs? Or mine? I couldn't see any other possibility. I resolved that I would care for my parents unto the end. But no way did I dream I would be caring for *thirty years*! The doctor said my mother defied medical opinion. They said my good caring must have kept her going so long!

What gave you strength throughout that time?
My faith in God. Every day He gives me strength.

Have you always believed in God?
Since age four when I went to Sunday school at the local Baptist church. Each night I would say prayers before sleep. I believe God gave me courage to cope as a carer. I have prayed when I crawled on my hands and knees up the stairs to bed. I would say God help me, I cannot do another day. It seemed humanly impossible to keep caring for two seriously ill people single-handed. But a new day would dawn and although the tasks remained the same, somehow I would find renewed strength. I could not have done this on my own; the strength was obviously given to me. A certain prayer that I had learned at school gave me much strength throughout my caring years.

ST IGNATIUS' PRAYER FOR GENEROSITY

Lord, teach me to be generous.
Teach me to serve you as you deserve;
to give and not to count the cost,
to fight and not to heed the wounds,
to toil and not to seek for rest,
to labour and not to ask for reward,
save that of knowing that I do your will.
                    – *St Ignatius Loyola 1491–1556*

Did you never once lose your faith in God?
Never God. I lost my faith in people. When my caring role was at its peak my father was so ill it was impossible to leave him with my mother for even an hour so I could get to church as usual. I was a pianist for the church for twenty years. When I stopped attending church, the church soon forgot about me. Also my experience was that, when my mother developed Alzheimer's and was no longer recognised as a human being with a spiritual need, even the Ministry failed her. After my father's funeral, never once did the minister come

to see her. I do not attend church now, yet God remains close, a true friend. I now see that being a Christian is not about going to church on a Sunday. It is about what you are as a person. Having a thought for people in sickness and in health. It does not cost anything to show a little compassion.

Did you accept your role as a carer easier because you believed that is what God had in store for you?

It could be argued that yes this is what God had in store for me. Perhaps God saw me as the best person to fulfil the role? There were times when my parents' health did improve and I would think okay it's safe to move out, set up home on my own and find employment but before the plan could be put into action another crisis would hit. It would have been inhuman to leave them in those circumstances. So perhaps this was God's choice for me?

Past caring, I had to find a new purpose in life. A new identity. I asked God for strength and some ideas. I prayed for my new future to bring me happiness and fulfilment and a sense of peace.

Has it?

It truly has. It's been bumpy getting here, though.

What made a difference?

Two things stand out. In 1989 my mother's health had deteriorated so much that all she could do unaided was breathe. I knew that she could not survive much longer. Questions haunted me. What would happen to me after she died? How would I survive financially? What would I do with my life? What would I be capable of doing with my life? How many working years would be left for me to build up National Insurance contributions? Over the years I had lost myself. Lost my identity, confidence, social life and income.

I would now urge all carers to hang onto their job no matter if they have to pay out every penny to bring care in. It is terribly difficult to get back into the workplace once you have had a long time out.

As it was, I knew that I could continue working in a caring environment but desperately needed something different.

In 1989, whilst still a carer, I saw an advertisement in my local newspaper for the University of Wales, a Diploma in Social Studies – this was an access course to further education on completion. The course ran two mornings a week for a year. Crossroads Care

Attendants sat with my mother only one morning per week. The college made a concession and allowed me to attend one morning per week over two years. And Crossroads kindly gave me an extra hour. So at the grand age of forty-nine I started college. It was tough being a sole carer and studying but I stuck at it.

During the second year of the diploma my mother died. In my grief, I couldn't care less about keeping going and completing the course. I almost gave up, then thought hang on, Mary, it gives you somewhere definite to go every Friday. For that reason I kept at it and passed the exams. I had an excellent course tutor who took a personal interest in my circumstances. The tutor felt I was capable of further study. Looking back now, had I not been on that diploma course when my mother died, goodness knows where I might have ended up. I would have been totally lost. This is why I would encourage carers and past carers to become involved in learning. Community Education offers a wide range of subjects for all ages. Had I not been involved on the diploma course, I may never have discovered I was capable of academic study, never have gone on to do a degree. Most of all, I would never have had someone there to encourage me. Believe in me.

The second turning point was when *I* began to believe in me. Up to that point I had been keeping going but on very shaky ground. Many times I thought of giving up, believing that I was not good enough, listening too much to what others thought of me. But in the second year of the degree course we had to study a module in counselling. This part of the course involved us, the students, taking a good look at our lives and the choices we had made. I began to see things about my past in a new light. I began to see the role I played in my life. I can now look back on caring and see that the door was there. I could have walked through it and gone. It took guts to stay and guts to go. In the end, love won. I loved my mother and father and so I chose to look after them. Yes, it was at a great personal cost. Yet, in a sense, what a privilege it was to care for a loved one until death – to be able to. I now feel proud to have been a carer but at the time I was so run-down I thought I was useless. Worthless.

I see now the remark the neighbour made about having nothing to offer, the remark that hurt me so, was perhaps not so much her being deliberately nasty, but rather because I was listening to her through such low self-esteem. *I* thought I had nothing to offer. Now if people say negative things to me it washes right off. I believe in me, regardless. It has taken a long time to get to this point, though. Re-building confidence has been, and is, an on-going journey.

Counselling taught me acceptance of my past. I learned that it is not bad to let go. Nothing anyone can do or say can change the past. We can only change the present, the future. Right now is where you, I, have power. If I do not like the way something is today I can do something about it. The past is gone. The day I fully accepted my past exactly as it was, is the day I began to live again. And in accepting my past I learned to accept me for me. I was able to say look, this is who I am, this is what I've been doing, this is it. Me.

You mean look back with no regrets?

It's more acceptance of how it was. It's seeing that bitterness or saying 'if only' or 'I wish' doesn't help. Oh yes, you have to grieve, I'm not saying don't grieve. Grief is natural, healthy. Unresolved grief makes it very difficult to move on. Acceptance is accepting that you cannot change how things were.

Like, when I was a young woman I longed to get married and have five sons. My father would laugh and say "Oh yes, have you put the order in with God?" Then when caring for my parents, age twenty-six I made a decision; that I was not going to have children after all. There is a supposed link with Alzheimer's and Down's Syndrome. I thought I'm not going to bring a child into the world just to satisfy my need. Not when there is a chance that my child may suffer like my parents were suffering. I did not think that fair.

So you see I would have loved children if things had been different. But they were not different. And the healthy acceptance of this is what allows me to be able to live fully today.

Same with a relationship. When caring there was not a moment to think about sex or relationships. Goodness, I did not even have a social life! That is not to say I would not have liked a relationship if things had been different. They weren't.

I knew that I could have ended up a very bitter and lonely person. But what good is that? That would have been such a waste of what was left of my life. Through learning more about me I saw that I could change my attitude to my past. My perspective on it.

Acceptance even comes in when I look back and see that my stubborn streak perhaps hindered me when caring. I would not ask for support until I was desperate. I probably made things harder for myself at times. But being stubborn has also been helpful in re-building my life. I have achieved a lot. Risen from the ashes. I am proud of me. I accept me, past and present. That is not to say I do not look back and see that I could have asked for more support earlier. I look back. I see it. I do not beat myself up over it.

Accepting my past gave me a new outlook. I began to look to the future, rather than dwell on what had been. I saw that the future could be better than what I had. That motivated me. This desire to better myself, my life. It gave me a new purpose. Through education I developed personally and academically. I set goals, then moved the goals and stretched myself a little more. It was hard at first, very hard, but then it became fun, challenging in a good way.

When you wrote to me in 1998 you said although you had your degree and your counselling certificate you still could not get paid work. What changed?

I was doing voluntary work for the Right Crowd, an educational organisation for people with learning disabilities. I had been working there some time. A paid post became vacant. Nobody spoke to me about applying for it. I sat there thinking, oh well, I must be invisible. I can do it but nobody offers me a pay packet. Then I thought okay, no good sitting here just thinking about it, Mary. The job was to teach assertiveness skills and independent living to young people with special needs! So I went to the person in charge and said I hear this job is going and I just want to let you know I am interested. I believe that I can do it. That month I got my first pay packet in thirty years. I have learned that in life sometimes you have to ask for what you want. Having that first paid position moved mountains. More teaching positions have come my way. I now have an income, improved self-esteem, a job and life I love. I kept faith, kept focussed, even on the hardest days, that everything would work out.

Tell me about some of your hardest days, caring and past caring.

After my father died it was awful. I had no chance to grieve as I was immersed in twenty-four hour care for my mother, a mammoth task. Her physical frailty left her non-weight bearing and the Alzheimer's meant that there was little communication between us. One day I took her to the cemetery and asked her if she liked the stone I had chosen for Dad. "So this is where he is," was her reply, "I wondered where he had gone to." I felt so sad. I missed my father terribly. For months after his death I felt physically sick. Although his health had been poor he had a good spirit, we could have a laugh, a conversation, a debate. Then he was gone. No time to grieve as caring took all my energy. Sometimes my mother would be so agitated I would have to pace the house with her right through the night. I was there with her every step of the way as she slowly descended into a vegetative state. On top of this came financial worries. I didn't know how we would cope. With the loss of my father's state pension and his occupational pension (it was not paid to widows) and with hefty bills (laundry was an on-going chore and our heating on constantly as my mother was prone to hypothermia) I did not see how we would manage. We did though by cutting down on perks such as cream cakes when I went shopping. The last two years of my mother's life were horrendous. I believe in living wills. I would rather be dead than go through what my mother did.

I remember saying to the doctor 'what a blessing', when my mother died. I was glad she was at peace and free from pain. I said I'm not going to grieve. Six months later, I was shopping in one of the large stores in town and after paying for the goods I turned with the bags as though to place them on the handles of the wheelchair. It suddenly struck me; I no longer had a mother. I was weepy for weeks. The GP said this was nature's way. The grief, whether I wanted it or not, was emerging. But it seemed that no-one was prepared to comfort me. I wondered where all the people were that came to the funeral, who said 'we are here for you' but never made further contact. One day I was truly desperate to talk to someone. I phoned a friend. They said they were too busy to talk that day, they would call another day. When I tried to talk about how I felt, people would change the subject. Soon I learned to keep things to myself.

Another tough time was when I started university. It felt awkward being amongst people again. I had lost the art of small talk, of socialising. A lot of the students would end up sitting together and I'd end up sitting on my own. I felt so sad and lonely. It may sound funny but at those times I longed for my old life back. I see now it was just a period of re-adjustment. Any change is a challenge. After a few months I finally made a friend and life became sweeter.

And you have a relationship now. How did that come about?

A friend asked me to help out with a Scouts do at the Church. I nearly didn't go, couldn't be bothered, then decided, Oh, I'll go. She had also asked Tony to help out. He used to be at school, in the year above me. I liked him way back then. We said hello and chatted a bit. His mother had died not long before too. He asked if I fancied meeting up again and we arranged to meet the following week. We went for a meal in town.

So was your friend playing Cilla Black all along?

She denies it, totally. Tony and I joke, we say what on earth are our mothers doing up there?

And romance blossomed?

Yes, it took a while. We were just friends for five years. After thirty years of not having a relationship I did not want to rush things! No, really, it was scary. When Tony went to give me a hug I would automatically tense up. Touch was so unfamiliar. It felt strange having someone close after thirty years on my own. After Mum died I didn't expect to meet anyone, I didn't go looking. I mean, you've gone without for so long. It took time. Time to build trust, friendship. We've been together eleven years now. He is a good man. It's so lovely to have someone special

* * *

Sex

Relationships past caring can be a scary prospect. Carers, through the demands of the caring life, get used to being self-contained, isolated, their 'own person'.

I spoke to men and women who, past caring, had been scared to get close, who gave intimacy a body-swerve.

> After my father died I found having lots of sex helped. But I wasn't interested in an emotional commitment. Sex gave me a sense of life after being surrounded by death. Sex acted as a release for the adrenaline that had built up over the years. I have read soldiers, both men and women, returning from war (or other traumatic event), experience something similar.
>
> *(Peter from London, thirty-nine, a past carer for his father, mother and sister)*

> I moved back from London where I was working in Television to care for my Mum. I'm an only child, my father died many years ago. I cared for Mum for two and a half years. I didn't have a relationship or a social life in that time. I felt like I might go crazy. I masturbated a lot! It reminded me of being a teenager back in my old bedroom! After Mum died, I just wanted to get out of my mind. Most nights I'd go to gay bars drink, flirt, drink more. I met lots of men but because I was out my mind half the time I didn't connect with them. Didn't connect with anyone. It was a lonely, sad shocking time. I hurt myself and others. In the end, I went into a residential therapy centre to tackle my destructive behaviour. And I got to see that what I was really in was shock.
>
> *Michael, a forty-six year old gay man from Glasgow*

Voices echoed each other.

> I date and sleep with men but I refuse to make a commitment. Perhaps I've been so hurt by grief in the past I'm afraid to be happy? Caring has made me not want to share my life and that makes me sad. But it's so difficult to see my future with another person as I like the independence and no longer having to do this, fetch that etc. I've been given back my wings and I want to fly free. Could you imagine if that person got ill? I just couldn't do it all over again.

Shock causes many couples who have devotedly cared for a beloved child or elderly relative to split up when the caring has ended. Having been bonded by a common aim, in grief they may turn away from one another, disconnect from one another, sometimes even blame each other.

Debbie Harry, the singer from Blondie, put her singing career on hold to care for her boyfriend Chris Stein when he was diagnosed with a life-threatening illness. For almost four years she slept in a cot bed in his hospital room so she could be with him night and day. Thankfully, he got better. After he recovered they split up, but remain friends. In an interview afterwards she said, "I didn't know who I was anymore. I was really lost and very, very depressed. Chris was trying to recover and I was trying to recover. There just wasn't room in the relationship for two recoveries."

* * *

Sole carers suffer from sensory deprivation. Touch. Cuddles. Whispers. Kisses. Warm skin. Hugs. Sweat. They may start off with the same desires as everyone else, but as the years pass and they remain stuck in the house caring, unable to go out and meet people, build a social life, a sex life, how do they cope?
Many people were a wee bit shy when I suggested talking about sex.

> "We've never been asked about that side of things before. We've thought about it, often, every day sometimes, but nobody has ever asked us about it.
>
> It's taboo. Tucked away. Out of sight. You don't bring it up. You ignore it. Repress it. You talk about everything else but you don't talk about <u>sex</u>!"

They said even carers groups and the official caring organizations didn't talk about... "Y'know…"

I said, "I want to talk about sex. Do you mind?"

"It'll be a relief," they said.

> Down there? You switch it off. You know you're not going to be able to use it for a long time. Problem is, you can't remember how to switch it back on. It hibernates. Sometimes it dies off completely. Yes, that's how it feels. Dead. You're too tired to care. Too tired to think about it. You're too exhausted at night to do anything else but sleep anyway. Just call me Sister Maria! Watch sexy films. You turn the sound down low and hope your mother doesn't hear. DIY. I'm a DIY expert. At first it's a nightmare. Then you learn to live with it. Or rather, live without it.

But for carers like Gordon, caring for his wife with advanced MS, the 'mind-numbing sexual frustration' brings daily mental anguish. He told me: "I love and care for my disabled wife but the truth is I dream of having a purely sexual relationship with someone else every single day."

When I write to him to ask if I can use his comments and that I will change his name to protect his privacy he bravely writes back: 'If you wish to use my correct name in full I would not be offended or embarrassed in any way at all. There is absolutely no point in accusing others of avoiding the true reality of caring (by not addressing the sexual needs of the carer) and then hiding myself behind another name.'

Susan from Cumbria shares her story here because she says:

I needed to talk about sex. I was lucky to find someone who understood. I know others need to talk about sex and are not so lucky. My advice is not to bottle it up but speak up. That's the only way we will change things. Under our clothes we're all the same.

My husband was diagnosed with Parkinson's (and latterly dementia) whilst I was in my thirties. We had a young family, a bright future to look forward to. The news devastated us but we kept positive and took one day at a time.

This disease is a slow-burn disease with a gradual loss of physical ability. At the beginning it was not too bad because we could continue in some way with a sex life but as my husband's mental and physical condition worsened our relationship moved from that of man and woman to more of a mother-son relationship. My husband required more and more care. Feeding, washing, lifting. At night I would have to undress him, toilet him, wipe his bottom. It's just … when I got into bed beside him, I didn't feel aroused to have sex. Not because I didn't love him. I did love him. But when he was well enough to try to have sex, it would be such an effort and would end up so unsatisfactory. In Parkinson's the body spasms involuntary and well … you can imagine. In the end the thought of sex became a turn-off for me. But he would still want to try. I now feel guilty that I didn't try harder. But at the time … I suppose … I just longed for a sex life that would leave me satisfied as a woman. I longed for a man who was stronger and more powerful and who could take care of me physically. That's what I had lost. The feeling of being a woman.

Over the years I was terribly lonely. I envied healthy couples. To lie at night next to someone you love but can no longer make love to is the worst kind of loneliness.

As my husband's health deteriorated he would spend two weeks in hospital and four weeks at home. Around this time he said to me one day "If you ever want to have a friend, just don't tell me."

I got very low. I needed to talk to someone but there seemed nowhere to turn. You don't want to tell friends because you sound disloyal. You don't want to hurt your husband, you feel so bad because it's not their fault. We are all helpless against the horrors of disease. My husband had to deal with losing his sexual identity too. Nobody wants to upset anyone. So sex remains a hush-hush subject.

Then, at my GP surgery one day, I suddenly began pouring my heart out. I told him how tired and frustrated I was. My GP was fabulous. He said, "What you need to do is give yourself a day that is all yours. Be a bit selfish. Just devote that day to yourself, your needs. And have you ever considered a purely physical relationship with someone?"

I was amazed. There was no judgement. I still think that men have an easier time. Y'know. If a man has a purely sexual affair people say, "Oh well, he's a man." But for a woman … it doesn't feel so acceptable in our society. It's as if women should still be just carers and mothers. But women need sex too.

My GP then referred me to a counsellor – a clinical psychologist. I was feeling desperate but also so guilty just considering this course of action. The counsellor was understanding and really helped to guide me through these guilty feelings – and encouraged me to do something about my situation.

I plucked up courage and called an old friend from my hometown. I knew he was on his own as his wife had died from cancer some years previously. I thought 'he is probably lonely too'. I asked if he would like to meet up for lunch.

We did and thereafter we met one day a week – that was all.

After all these years it was lovely and exciting to be dressing-up and going out somewhere and feeling attractive again.

That one day a week was heaven – an oasis and an escape from the daily drudgery of caring.

I became more relaxed, more energised. We gradually progressed from companionship to a physical relationship.

The thought of abandoning my husband never entered my mind. Nobody knew, apart from my three children. They understood, they supported me, looked after their Dad so I could have that day. One day a week was sufficient. Yes, I did fall a little in love with my friend as he did me. But my friend knew and accepted my situation. He would never have done anything to hurt my husband. Nor would I.

There was guilt – oh yes, the guilt was still there, but in a way I felt relieved that I had done something to help myself. I had seen many carers become ill under the stress of caring. I could not have gone on much longer without something giving. A part of me had died and I had reclaimed it. I had taken care of me and in doing so was able to take better care of my husband. Having that relief of physical and sexual tension saved me. It gave me back my sense of being a healthy normal woman. And my GP is delighted I have not become a long-term patient of his.

Ironically, my friend fell ill and died a few years before my husband. And although this was of course a very hard time, what I had gained in terms of energy and life from our relationship helped me go on to care devotedly for my husband until his death.

* * *

As humans we crave not only physical affection, but also companionship. If we don't have a companion, a friend we can talk to, we feel lonely. If carers are lucky they can talk openly to the person they are caring for but illness and pain can make people short-tempered and grumpy. There may be irritation on both sides. The love is there the liking is not. And for those caring for someone with a disease like Alzheimer's, they have the added distress of witnessing their companion 'disappear'. It is important to have a friend we can talk to openly.

Audrey, from Essex, is eighty-four years old. She writes: "I cared for my husband who had a stroke for twenty-four years. Now my husband is long dead, as are most of my friends. I can no longer drive so rarely leave the house. If I did not talk to the cat, I'm sure I would lose the power of speech."

Monica tells me: "I felt I needed to be in touch with people who understood exactly what it was like. Through an ad in the *Carer* magazine I am now in contact with two male carers, one of whom has been wonderfully supportive. He did not know my mother so I feel I can talk to him honestly without feeling disloyal. I can talk to him and know he understands exactly what I am on about."

But how, after years caring, do people meet people?

I asked a group of healthy adults who had never been involved in caring where they had met their partners and the most popular answer was: - through work.

WANTED: Desperately seeking Past Carers for … Past Carers!

Well, why not? I thought. What about a companion/dating club for past carers? And then …

Deep in the land of Nod much too late one Sunday morning, I was awakened by a phone call.

"That you Audrey?"

I recognised the voice of Alan, a carer I had interviewed some time before who had looked after his wife Alice for fifteen years.

"Did I wake you?"

"No, no ,"I rasped, my voice uncannily like Hannibal Lecter.

"I just wanted to let you know … there's a happy ending to the story."

A chuckle.

"I got married again."

An Interview with Alan and Sheila

The first thing that struck me when I saw Alan* again was how much younger he looked than the last time I had seen him. He positively glowed. And it wasn't just from the heat of the log fire in the lovely, new home that he shares with his wife of three years, Sheila. This was down to love. Marriage, dare I ask? ...

Yes. We have sex.

Alan is laughing.

I'm seventy-three now and Sheila's sixty-five. People say 'Oh, isn't it nice to have a companion for your old age?' I think people think we got together for purely practical reasons. But there's romance! At our ages we re-discovered a physical relationship as well as companionship after all the barren years.

How did you two meet?

Alan: We were both doing voluntary work at Voice of Carers Across Lothian. We were both carers at the time. Alice, my first wife, was in long-term hospital care and Sheila's husband Bob was between home and respite care. We became friends. We were both carers, and had been for many years, for spouses with a debilitating illness. Sheila cared for twenty-six years. We could support each other because we understood what it was like for one another. We were never romantically involved with each other whilst our spouses were still alive. In fact, it never crossed either of our minds. We were simply work-mates who had a lot in common, who were working together to promote something we passionately believed in; raising awareness and support of carers. In fact, I met Sheila's husband a couple of times when I dropped her home after VOCAL duties. I never dreamt one day that I would be her husband. At that time our heads were filled with how best to care for our spouses. There was no time or energy to think of anything else. We just gave each other advice and help where we could."

So ... tell us how romance came around ?

Sheila: Our spouses died within six months of one another in 1996. This was a very tough time and Alan and I gave each other a lot of support but on a purely friendship level. Cups-of-tea-and-

---

* Alan's first interview is on page 77

sympathy type of thing. We were both very involved in the work of VOCAL, both of us were doing public speaking about Caring to all sorts of organisations. Public speaking is nerve-wracking and Alan would support me and I him. So we were very good friends for about three years before anything romantic happened.

The first sign of romance came when Alan asked me to join him up North. He has a time-share near Loch Rannoch. I was quite thrilled to be asked because I did like him. But I was scared. Although we got on well as friends, we mostly went out socially because of work commitments or because one of us had an invitation to a 'couply' thing. For those occasions, it's nice to have a male friend you can call upon or vice versa to be your escort, y'know, balance the numbers. So although we were friends, we hadn't really gone out together socially on an obvious date ... I panicked a little and thought oh what if we don't really get on and it's just the two of us together for a week? So I said I would go up for one day and one night.

That way, if we weren't really suited, I could run home fast.

Alan, weren't you scared too ... you know the thing of ... don't spoil a good friendship?

Alan: Yes, I was scared. I had always thought of Sheila as just a friend but then I started to have these thoughts creeping in. I started to miss her when I didn't see her. I began to think of her more as a woman than just a friend. But I didn't know how to tell her and I didn't know what she was thinking so yes, I was scared of spoiling things ... I wanted to make it clear that it wasn't just a casual invitation, that I really wanted Sheila to join me up North, but I didn't want to sound too heavy. I wanted to be cool but not too cool. When she said okay I'll come up for one day and one night, I was a bit disappointed she didn't want to come up for the week, but I thought still, it's a good sign.

And romance blossomed that trip?

Alan: Oh no. We were terribly polite. We each had our own rooms and slept in them. I was scared of messing things up, scared of rejection so I thought take it easy Alan. I was the perfect gentleman."

Sheila: I came back thinking oh well, he's not made a move so he **does** only want to be friends. I was a bit disappointed! But at least I knew we did get on, just the two of us. We'd had a good time together, a laugh. I even got Alan snorkelling in the swimming pool.

Alan: I forced myself. I was scared she would think I was a wimp otherwise.

Sheila: So when Alan asked me, two months later, to go to Spain for a fortnight I thought okay, I know he only thinks of me as a friend but we do get on well, so why not?

Alan: … and all the time. I was sitting there fretting … how on earth am I to tell her I want it to be more and not spoil things if she just thinks of me as a friend? I had lost so much confidence with women. I had not had a physical relationship for sixteen years.

Sheila: So we went to Spain and we had our own rooms.

Alan: And we slept in our own rooms and everything was all very proper until.

Sheila: Half way through the week … we were just about to go out for dinner and we were having drinks on the patio when Alan said.

Alan: Where do you want to go from here?

Sheila: And I turned it around and said. Where do you want to go from here?

Alan: And I said … I would like it to go further.

Sheila: And I said so would I. And at dinner we held hands. And do you know how lovely it is to hold hands after having no physical affection for years? Just to hold hands became so, so sacred. Because, in the end, as a carer you may still be married and you may still love your husband or wife but the illness can rob you of physical intimacy. You can no longer hold each other because it's too sore, too uncomfortable, or, in cases like Alzheimer's, the person withdraws physically. You're like a plant without water. You wither. You lose touch with your skin, body. So to hold someone's hand again it's like … I can't describe it.

Alan: And when we came back to the apartment we held each other close … and then shared the same bed.

Sheila: We were both nervous and anxious to please.

Alan: So nervous that things didn't go quite as planned.

Sheila: And we laughed about it. We could laugh about it because we knew each other so well. We joked about it and said don't worry, that'll come in time and we just lay together and it was so, so beautiful and warm to feel so close to someone again.

Alan: Over the years of caring, I had physically cut off from my sexuality. I had poured every ounce of physical energy into doing the work of VOCAL and campaigning for carers. It was physically and emotionally a lonely life. Yes, every now and again, sitting at home reading the newspaper my eye would stray to the adverts for saunas and for a second I'd think oh … what if? … but then a 'sensible' part takes over. I suppose the stigma of it doesn't help. I used to be a Church elder! I'd think … what if someone saw me arriving, leaving? And I'd put it out of my mind, try to focus on something else. So, being with a woman again was a bit like diving into a freezing swimming pool. Exciting but quite a shock.

Sheila: We got engaged that week and our friends said they weren't surprised. The great thing was that all our children were delighted. I have three sons and a new grandson and Alan has a son and a daughter and four grandchildren. I think when children are around illness and caring they often grow up to be more caring towards others themselves. We are lucky. We had the blessing of all our children to go ahead and get married. And they said to us, c'mon now, it's time that you two did something just for yourselves.

Alan: And so we cut back on some of our work commitments with VOCAL and we signed up for watercolour classes in painting. We're still involved in work for carers but we're also doing fun things for ourselves now.

Sheila: And we did up this house together. We didn't want for one of us to move into the other's house. We decided to start afresh and it feels right.

Was there any guilt, feelings of disloyalty toward the memory of Bob or Alice?

Both: No. We recognised that that part of our life was over. It doesn't mean we no longer have the fondest memories or love still for our first husband and wife. But we recognised that chapter had ended. We could either stay stuck or move on. Life brought us together. We felt blessed that we had the chance to make a new beginning at this stage in our lives.

Life brought you together but isn't it true that you had to help it along a bit?

Alan: Yes. Life brings opportunities to us but we have to recognise them and take steps too … even though I was uncertain of what may or may not happen, even though I was scared of rejection, I had to take a chance, risk making my feelings known.

Sheila: If you'd never suggested the trip up North or the trip to Spain, we might still be sitting in our houses on our own …

Alan: We were lucky how things turned out. At seventy-three years old, I feel like I'm living again. As a carer I felt only half-alive.

Sheila: Me too.

Doesn't your experience of being a carer put you off wanting to care again?

Sheila: Well since we married a couple of our family have been quite ill. Having each other has enabled us to cope, we give each other a lot of support, just like in the old days.

But what if one of you has to care again full-time if the other falls ill?

Alan: It didn't even cross our minds. If and when it happens we'll deal with it. Life's too short to worry.

* * *

Memory - The Present

As I walk back from Alan and Sheila's new house, Edinburgh Castle lights the sky, brightens black wet streets. I love the sight of the Castle, majestic, way up there, protector, Carer of the City. As I walk, a thought, a question, is niggling me.

What is it that makes some people – carers – recover much better – is that the right word? – than others. What I'm trying to say is: what is it that allows some people to go on to create some kind of purpose in a new world, whilst others remain firmly stuck?

I had interviewed many carers who had gone on to create a new life.

But what of all the letters I had received where people had not? Letters full of anger, bitter, blaming.

I had been one of those souls that seemed to be stuck, lost for ages. I remained unforgiving of this unfair world. Obsessed with the suffering of life as opposed to the celebration. Never allowing myself - through feelings of guilt or undeserving - to know happiness or joy. Instead I repeated the same script over and over. Life's shit. Nothing lasts. Why bother? Don't get close … I remained detached, unable to connect to others. Efforts at career or relationships seemed to go so far, then fall apart. For years I had felt trapped in feelings of futility, of failure. A maze of dead ends. But then doesn't even running into a dead end tell us something?

When I was a child, my parents told me about the secret path that winds up and up and up and up on what appears to be the Castle's sheer impassible rock-face. I remember my amazement, upon hearing how, centuries ago, soldiers climbed up this path in the dead of night and so surprised the enemy. As a child, I would stare really hard into the rock, thinking, how could you climb up that? It looked impossible.

"Why can't I see the path?" I'd bleat to Mum.

"Because you can't just see it," she said. "You have to search for it." Then she added: "Maybe it depends on where we're standing?"

I had intended to write this book as some kind of sharing of stories. But I came to be fascinated not just by the stories but what lay behind the stories. What meaning the story-teller gave to the story. How they had chosen to make sense of what did – or didn't – happen.

In the light of hearing others, I looked at my own story again. What had I decided – what meaning had I given to having been involved in caring for my parents in my teens and twenties? I watched. Listened. Looked.

I believed as a child that if we looked long enough up at the Castle rock, perhaps, at some point in the dense black, we may see a crack of light. If we are too close, that may be all we see. But if we are far enough away, we may see more.

More moments of illumination.

As I looked at my own story of past caring, slowly, slowly, patterns began to emerge. How, as an adult, I remain, in many ways, as helpless as a child, unable to cook, unable to drive, stuffing bills under cushions, even remaining unable to work the computer I use to write this. I have to go running to the library staff every two minutes to ask: "Please, can you do this for me, sort that, copy this bit here."

So remaining like a child I believe … what? I can avoid the responsibility of caring again? So I may, in a sense, remain free?

But then, by avoiding taking on some kind of responsibility, don't I miss out on many more aspects of what it is to be truly free? To get in the car and go for a drive. To pay for this or that without worrying where the next pay-packet is coming from (past caring, I haven't had a regular job for years.) Certainly, at first there was the burn-out, the exhaustion, but then … did it become an excuse, self-justification? 'I cared so I can't'.

And what of my relationships with men? The pattern that emerged that first summer past caring may have been exactly right for then. But it – I – had got stuck in the groove, years later, still afraid of having to care for another, either emotionally or physically. Afraid of losing myself. Of being hurt. Of course, I still got hurt. (As if by saying 'I can't care', I could keep myself safe.)

This fear had made me demanding of men. Past caring, I had a notion that love was about giving and expecting nothing back in return. For isn't this the relationship between the carer and the cared for? And isn't that about love? I forgot - or deliberately overlooked? Most healthy adult relationships are based on tit for tat, give and take, a partnership. And isn't it by being able to give both to ourselves and others that we may grow? Discover new things?

So as I walked beneath the Castle, a thought occurred to me.

Yes, it is true that being involved in caring for my parents during my teens and twenties has made me want to defend my freedom. But isn't freedom about choice as opposed to entrapment? Isn't it about running in the gardens as opposed to crouching, arrows-at-the-ready, in the watch-tower? And so … being free could mean one thing or another … depending on where I'm standing?

And 'nothing lasts' could mean one thing or the other … depending on the angle I'm looking at it? Life is impermanent. Everything we have is taken from us by death. So, if everything we have is taken away by death, then why bother starting anything? Or, if everything we have will be taken away by death, what have I got to lose? I can enjoy today rather than, through fear, deny myself? And if I share myself today, is that also destroyed by death? Or could sharing myself perhaps be a way of saying look, you cannot take this away, because I have already given it away?

Above me, the sky and Castle are floodlit; magical, fairy-tale like. A battleground, a fortress? How closely connected is the potential for creation and destruction.

The self-help books had told me that good can come from suffering. I thought: perhaps it is not so much that good can come from suffering but rather we humans have to *create* the good from suffering. For what is the alternative?

Somewhere, far above me, the path. I cannot see it. I must simply trust that it is there. If I choose.

* * *

When tragedy strikes we struggle to make sense of it. At the time it does not make any sense. We search, regardless. Later, if we are lucky, we may catch glimpses, tiny insights as they are revealed to us.

One man who has been searching for the past three decades is Lord Swraj Paul. Lord Paul's younger daughter, Ambika, died of leukaemia, aged four and a half.

I had seen Lord Paul, now seventy years of age, on the *Esther* show. He was one of five millionaires who were being interviewed about how they had made their money. Lord Paul seemed to me to possess a special humility, humanity. During the show he talked briefly of his daughter and the effect her death had had on his life.

I wrote to Lord Paul requesting an interview for this book. As I posted the letter I thought, 'Oh, he'll probably not respond, he'll be too busy.'

I met with Lord Paul the following week in his London office. In the flesh he was as warm as on television. I immediately felt at ease. So at ease, that at one point during the interview, I cried.

In response to a question I had asked him, Lord Paul said to me, "Audrey, I am going to give you the same advice I would give to my children. I am now going to talk to you just as I would talk to my children."

His words moved me. For in them I knew my loss. I knew how much I had missed, would always miss, having the care and advice of my parents and the gaping void that leaves in my life. In that moment I envied Lord Paul's children, just as I have caught myself, over the years, envying my friends and the way their parents care for them, look after them, still, in the unique way that only parents do for their children. No matter how old their 'children' are.

The relationship, the bond between child and parent, parent and child, is so unique that nothing can replace it. It is not the love of a lover, or a dear friend, or any other relative. It is beyond that.

And I saw how, since my parents died, I have been searching for that kind of care. How I have longed to be looked after in such a way. It is no coincidence that I enjoy the company of older men and women. And when they talk of their children, yes, I feel envious, feel like saying, please, would you like to adopt me?

I have searched but never found this kind of unconditional care that exists between parent and child. How can I? My parents are dead. And to expect a lover to be a parent substitute only leads to disaster. Oh yes. I see that now!

When Lord Paul said to me, "Audrey, I am now going to talk to you as I would talk to one of my children," I found myself crying. I thought, Oh no, I have come to interview Lord Paul about his daughter, yet I am the one crying. This is not the way it should be. But Lord Paul wasn't perturbed. As he passed me tissues he told me that he had been interviewed on television the other day and for two whole minutes he had been unable to speak, he was so upset. We laughed. He told me: "Do not worry about crying, Audrey, this is normal, this is natural. Your tragedy is more recent than mine. I would be more concerned if you were not crying, that would be abnormal."

In our culture, we have shied away from crying … someone cries and we say, "do not cry, don't be upset." We have made it a bad thing. Lord Paul made it a good thing. When we are in the company of another who allows us to simply be, these things happen.

Lord Paul and I talked about his search for meaning since Ambika's illness and death. On how this sequence of events had affected his being. At the time it didn't make any sense. For a small child to die before a parent is not the natural order of things. Unfortunately, it is the way of things. And for Lord Paul there are now glimpses in the puzzle that is life.

Lord Paul's Story

I was born and brought up in India. I was educated at Punjab University and then went on to study in the United States. Upon my return to India I got involved in the family business that my father had founded. And then of course, like all young men at that time, I got married. My lovely wife Aruna and I had four children. Our youngest was Ambika. Life was going quite well. I worked with my brothers in the family business, a conglomerate of hotels, steel and pharmaceuticals. Yes, life was very comfortable. What more can you have than a wonderful wife, lovely children, a flourishing business? Then tragedy struck. We came to know that Ambika was suffering from leukaemia.

At that time Ambika was two years old, an enchanting child, full of life. But she had been having spells of fever and listlessness. The doctors in Calcutta did not think it as anything too serious but a friend in New York, who happened to be a doctor, recommended some blood tests should be done. The tests were completed. The doctors in Calcutta said no, it wasn't leukaemia, but when I sent the same test results to my friend in New York, he said sadly this is leukaemia. He suggested we bring Ambika to the West for treatment. We decided to leave immediately for America. But Ambika's condition badly deteriorated. The specialist in Calcutta said she will never last the journey. So we decided to bring her to Britain instead.

We arrived in London in September 1966. Ambika was admitted to the Middlesex Hospital. We were told her illness was fatal. There was no cure.

What kept me going during this time and the further two years of caring for Ambika was the ultimate hope that she would be alright. Though deep down you know you are surely fighting a losing battle, you carry on with this hope, this belief that a miracle may happen. Unless you have that how can you look after them? I made sure she got all the best help, the best treatment possible and I existed on faith. Prayed for this miracle.

Both my wife and I came to London with Ambika. Work became secondary. This is where you see the strength of having a close family and a family business. For me, the greatest thing is the strength of the family. Fortunately, I have a wonderful family. My brothers and

I all lived together so leaving the other children behind was no hassle, my brothers and sister-in-law looked after them. We didn't have to worry about the business because that was all being taken care of. So we were here with only one thing to worry about – our little daughter. Aruna and I took turns to be at her bedside. My wife cared for her during the day, I at night. I would sit up in a chair. We would play, or pray together. In her childlike handwriting she would draft small letters to God to ask for blessings. She remained cheerful, innocent. Although the situation was torturous, we enjoyed every moment together.

On days when she was feeling better, I would take her to London Zoo. It was not far from our flat and the visit was a source of pleasure for her. She loved the animals. Some days she would seem quite well and our spirits would rise. Perhaps she would really be alright? But then, unfortunately, the sickness would return.

A dear friend in Delhi, a devout Catholic, wrote to me and said, 'Swraj, miracles happen at Lourdes. Why don't you take Ambika?' So we took her. At that time she was very weak, unable to walk. I was carrying her. I said to her, "Would you like to stand?" And … she stood. And then she was running around, running around, at Lourdes. And yes, it did seem in some small way like a miracle. But of course these things happen with leukaemia. Sometimes there is a remission and then the illness returns. When she fell ill again, as she entered the hospital for the last time she said she wanted to go back to Lourdes. In her mind, she associated Lourdes with being well. I told her okay, as soon as you are better, we will go. But unfortunately that was never to be.

Ambika died in April 1968, aged four and a half. Her passing left me shattered.

Immediately after cremating Ambika the family returned to India. (By this time our other children had joined us in London, my two sons and older daughter.) We returned to India, but I could not settle. I realised I wanted to go back to London, to be where Ambika had died. Also, the other children had been installed in school here and I did not really want to disturb them, they had gone through enough. I went to my brothers and told them this. They were fully supportive. Again, this is where you see the value of the family. I did not have to worry about working, or expenditure, because the joint family business supported us. These things as well as the family's emotional support helped me enormously. Without this, I would not have survived. This is where sometimes it is difficult to combine the philosophy in India with the thoughts of the West. Unfortunately, even in India, this kind of family strength does not operate so much anymore. But it does exist.

We returned to London, to the flat where we had lived with Ambika, the same flat we live in even today. I still could not concentrate. After Ambika died, my interest in life died. My wife and I were heart-broken, but she had far more energy than I. I have seen this not just in my wife, but in other women. They seem more able to cope with the pain. My wife's courage and determination to keep going helped me. In that way we became even closer, even stronger.

I lost all interest in work. Despair has a numbing effect.

What good is intelligence, money, status? What good is anything if it cannot save a loved one? Work was a struggle. Everything was a struggle.

I thought, Swraj, why do you want to live a life in which you have to struggle? What is the point? I thought, okay, let me accept this. Let me go. Let me instead concentrate on God. Let me pray, let me meditate. Let me read books on philosophy. On life.

So I entered Sanyas – withdrawal into a period of spiritual reflection and contemplation. I passed my days at home, praying, meditating, reading, thinking. The struggle then is to go through this practice and see what, if anything, is revealed. Many questions haunted me. I was searching for some kind of meaning to this inexplicable tragedy.

I read about others whose lives had been touched by tragedy. I came to know I was not the only one who had felt like this. A book that gave me much comfort and strength was Bertrand Russell's biography. (Russell's parents died when he was in early childhood.) As Bertrand's father was dying he wrote a letter to his own mother, Bertrand's grandmother. This letter affected me greatly. It showed me that I was not the only man who has had a problem. This realisation that I was not alone, this learning about others in similar situations, this helped me.

Another source of strength was my faith. I am Hindu. We believe in reincarnation. We believe every soul comes to the world with a purpose. So I came to think perhaps this girl came only for a message? Her life was so short she wanted to make something of it. She came with a message of life? Am I then perhaps too greedy because I wanted to keep her? Unfortunately, it is those left, that suffer more.

You go through all sorts of emotions, all sorts of thinking. One day, you think right, life has to move on and the next one, no, I can't move on. But after about eighteen months, a thought recurred, Swraj, you were not born to do nothing with your life.

Aruna and I decided to make a fresh start in Britain. I borrowed £5,000 from the bank and set up a company called Caparo. I did not want to ask my family for money although I knew they would have sent it immediately. I wanted to make it as tough as possible for myself. I didn't want to be comfortable. I wanted something that would take up all my energy, keep me busy, occupy me totally. It was a real test. Could I re-build a new life here in Britain?

The driving force in this decision was without question, Ambika. I believe she was, and is, driving me, guiding me, throughout my life. In Hinduism, we believe there is one God and then there are really the incarnations of God. My God may be Ambika. That doesn't mean that Ambika is God. It's personification in your own mind. What it means for you, what gives you your personal strength. I believe that Ambika lives within me and also, somewhere, out there. Like an angel, she watches over me. Because I tell you, opportunities have come, things have happened that could not have happened, except by something over which you have no control. An example … I have always had a thought, one day, if I have enough money, I will build something in memory of Ambika. When Ambika was alive, we rented a flat to be close to the Middlesex Hospital and we continued to live there after she died. I eventually bought that flat and the one next door. Then years later an opportunity came when the man who owned the building was looking to sell it. I told him, look, I know you would like to sell the building, I definitely would like to buy the building because I have something in mind. Whatever is the best offer you get I'll pay you £50,000 more. He never charged me the £50,000 more. He was a fair man. I bought the building and re-named it Ambika House. So you see this opportunity came and this kind of opportunity doesn't come even by design.

Then one day, in the early nineties, I was watching the television news and saw London Zoo is likely to close. They had run out of money. My only connection to the zoo was in the sixties when Ambika was ill and I would take her there to enjoy the animals. The thought occurred to me, if I can do something, let me save it. I wrote to them offering my help. They came up with a proposition for a new children's zoo that could survive on its own even if they may have to close the rest of the zoo. I said, okay, I will give you a million pounds. You make the best children's zoo in the world, most up-to-date. So you see it was a God-given opportunity, you cannot plan such things. Even if you start dreaming today I want to build something for Ambika, you have to find the land, find the place ... that is why I say that there is a message.

At the time, I wasn't sure what the message was. With hindsight, I see this girl came because she wanted to change my life completely. She brought me here to Britain. I would never have dreamt I would ever live in England. But this country has been very hospitable to me. My wife and I have had a good life here, with our family and grandchildren. After Ambika died, we were blessed with another child, a boy. I am a lucky man. God has been very kind.

Ambika came to this world with a message to change my life, this I am sure. And she remains a continuing memory. People talk about 'getting over someone'. But why should you want to shut this person out, leave this person you shared so much with, behind? I say let them be a part of your life now, today. Remember the joy they brought to you. Why would you want to forget? I think of Ambika every single day, she lives within me.

You ask me how can I be successful in the world of business and still remain a caring man? In my view, a businessman who is uncaring is not a businessman at all. You have to be a human being first and a human being last. In not just business, but every profession, whether it be teaching or law or whatever. Your duty is to do your job as best you can. If I am running a business my job is to try to ensure it is run successfully. Sometimes you have to make decisions that look uncaring on the day but your responsibility is that when you make those decisions it is in the interests of the whole business. You will make mistakes. You will make some correct decisions. But your success is not making all the right decisions, your success and hope is that you will make more right decisions than wrong ones. I never set out to be rich. I set out to run a successful business. All I can do is do what I do. But how things turn out is ultimately something over which I have no control.

So you see, in the end, Audrey, I will give to you the same advice I give to my own children. The thing to hang on to is faith. Whatever that faith may be. Don't let faith go out the window. Then you are finished. I believe there is definitely somebody above that monitors it all. Now whether they do a good job or a bad job may depend on your mental condition at the time. All you can do is do what you do. Beyond that, you are helpless.

One day I will die. I don't want to, but it will happen anyway. It's like the age-old story, everybody wants to go to heaven, but nobody wants to die. I have no control when, it may be today, it may be tomorrow, but my job until that time is to get on with what I do. There is a mystery to life that is beyond logic. What will happen will happen. We may wish it otherwise. The important thing is to keep faith that this is the way of life. We must ultimately trust it, though at the time, it makes no sense.

*   *   *

Care fact

A law was introduced recently, in October 2002, to allow carers to claim eight weeks Carers Allowance after the death of the person they cared for.

Prior to this law being introduced carers were expected to be available for work the day after their caring ended. On the day of death, all allowances the carer was entitled to stopped!

Carers allowance is currently £44.35 per week.*

Eight weeks at £44.35 makes a grand total of £354.80.

The work of informal carers save the Government and the tax-payer billions of pounds each year.

---

* As of April 2004

Communities

Lord Paul had said he was fortunate to be in a position to not have to worry about money when he took time off from work to recover from the loss of Ambika. He had said that without the emotional and financial support of his family he would not have survived.

I recalled once meeting the actress Phyllida Law, the mother of actresses Emma and Sophie Thompson. She had spent time caring for her own mother, making regular trips from London to the north of Scotland. She had sometimes missed out on work. I recalled her words: "I could not have survived financially if my girls had not helped me."

Many carers are not so lucky in the support, either financial or emotional, that they receive from their family. Families are more often than not scattered across the country. And so often, caring can cause a split in the family rather than a bond.

Being a carer cut me away from my siblings, who left me on my own to look after my stroke-ridden father. I had had the promise of help from two of my sisters and I still had friends in Leicester … Or so I thought. How do you convey the gut-wrenching loneliness of waiting for the door-bell to ring as you await the arrival of a promised visitor who does not come? A telephone that remains silent.

(Maria, Leicester)

I cared for my parents but my son and daughter hardly ever visit me. Yes, I do feel bitter. I don't think the younger generation will care like we did. They're too busy. Too selfish.

(Amber, Cornwall)

A caring life is isolating. To a carer the support of a caring (extended) family is immeasurable. It does not have to be direct help with the caring necessarily. (Although I'm sure that would be appreciated.) It could be running an errand, getting some shopping in, weeding the garden. It could be calling round with a treat to eat or a run in the car or hanging out the washing. It could be sitting with the ill person for a couple of hours whilst the carer has a snooze, a bath, goes to the hairdresser.

It may be the carer is too proud to ask. If families (and friends) are able to support each other, it not only spreads a load that threatens to crush one person carrying it alone, but also builds for a sense of community and belonging that so many people complain of having lost nowadays.

It is not surprising that there has been an increase in the number of people choosing to join together with other like-minded people and form their own communities. For these people living in a conventional set-up did not work. People came together and said; well, what can we do about this?

I decided to visit the world-famous community of Findhorn, situated on the magical shores of Findhorn Bay in the north of Scotland. In Findhorn members live either in their own ecologically-designed houses that they have bought, or they may share houses that belong
to the Foundation. Most members work outside the community. Some members work within it. People come from all over the world to lead courses on all kinds of spirituality. I noticed they had recently had a course called *Death, The Final Healing*, designed to help people lose their fear of dying and so live more fully; participants are encouraged to act out their own death.

I met with Barbara and Judith. I wanted to know – what happens when someone falls ill at Findhorn?

We have a group called Alanna. Alanna is a Celtic name that means 'carer of the soul'. Our group is a team of volunteers, both men and women, who come together to help care or offer assistance to a carer for someone who is ill or dying. We currently have around twelve core members, but numbers can fluctuate depending on a person's commitments. Those who are interested in becoming involved with Alanna let us know.

Likewise, if someone is in need of care they let us know. (We have a help-line number.) Then we will co-ordinate a rota of willing bodies. We've found that people are very willing to help out where they can. Our group is made up of all sorts of people, ex-teachers, lawyers, massage therapists, a researcher who worked at the House of Commons. Alanna members take it in turns to go to the house of the person who is ill and help with whatever needs doing. It may be simply doing the dishes or help with lifting or bathing or providing a ride to the hospital or … anything, really. If emergency help is needed during the night someone from Alanna will be on duty and the person in need will have their number. If someone needs help they just pick up the phone. That way caring, which is a huge strain for one person alone to manage, is never the responsibility of just one person.

If someone single falls ill and needs a serious amount of full-time care, we have a fund called the Elders Fund. Various community members give donations to this fund and we also organise fund-raising events. This Fund means that we can bring in a resident paid carer for the person who is ill and members of Alanna are also there to give support too.

We see caring as providing some kind of service to our community. We also have the experience of coming together to care. We come together to talk and share our feelings about what we are going through, what it means to us. We learn about ourselves from caring for the dying. We learn how real people are when they are dying. One lady used to talk of 'the tyranny of niceness'. She used to encourage her carers to be "real, true, honest. Mop up your own unfinished business. Don't wait until you are dying to relate to people." We are a team who support the dying person and each other. We try to help alleviate any fears the dying person may have, and in so doing we are brought up close with our own fears. We learn that death is the natural process of life. Our aim is to try to give the dying person the death they want. We don't judge. If they want to be taken to the beach, we'll take them. If they want to gather stones and rocks and sticks and place them all around the bed, we'll do this. We try to give them exactly what they want. We attempt to attend to their spiritual needs, whatever these needs are.

We also support the family. We help by arranging a burial or cremation in keeping with the person's wishes. After a death, because we have all cared in some way, no one is left alone in their grief unless they choose to be.

As well as Alanna, we also have groups of people from the community who visit an ill or housebound person to simply offer cheer for the spirit. Groups of people gather around the bedside and sing or do weaving or play music. One local lady, Judith, has just spent three years in America training in music Thanantology. This is the study of music for the dying. It had been found that harp music, played at certain vibrations and in time with the rhythm of the breath of the dying person, often assists the passing from one world to the next.

* * *

Whilst in Robertsbridge in Sussex visiting friends I was told about a community in the village called the Bruderhof, a Christian Community. My friends had recently moved into the area and were amazed at the unusual sight of these 'huge' families out for daily walks with the teenagers pushing the old people in massive wooden wheelchairs. I decided to see if I could talk to someone there. I met with Jutta. She explained:

> "With three hundred people living together with their own feelings, characters and backgrounds there is more than enough material for misunderstandings and differences of opinions. But they need not lead to tensions and conflicts if we are ready to open the door to one another in love and commitment."

People live and work on the community, which is self-sufficient. They have their own school, a farm, a publishing house and run several businesses making community educational playthings and equipment for people with disabilities. When members join the Bruderhof they donate all monies to the community. In return they are looked after for the rest of their lives.

"Invalid and elderly members are a treasured part of the community. Because the community (which includes members who are doctors and nurses) is like an extended family, we are often able to care for our sick and elderly at home. Wherever possible, birth and death takes place within the supportive atmosphere of the church community."

I became fascinated by the benefits that living on a community gave to carers. Of course, there are benefits and drawbacks in all kinds of lifestyles and when I mentioned to my friend about living on a community she screwed her face up in horror: "But everybody would know your business!"

"But," I said to my friend, "imagine if you were an exhausted carer, imagine you could just knock on your neighbour's door and say 'Excuse me, do you mind washing my dishes?' Wouldn't that be great?"

I thought, people could organize this within their own neighbourhoods, couldn't they? I recalled how Roald Dahl had trotted round his village asking for volunteers to help look after his wife Patricia Neal after her stroke. He got together a list of willing bodies. None of these people had any formal qualifications in 'caring'. Yet they did a terrific job (and one of those neighbours went on to write several books about the experience). And couldn't a street or two within a city become a village? Why shouldn't the impossible be possible?

Care Fact

Nearly six out of ten people give up paid employment to care.

Evidence shows that three in five of the population will at some stage take on the caring role for an ill loved one and many of us will be carers several times throughout our life.

Almost one in five carers cut down on their own food to survive financially when caring.

More than two out of three of the seven million carers in the UK worry most, or all of the time about finances.

As the train snaked out of London's Paddington station and headed west, winding its way along the Thames where I had sunk, many years before, into retreat, I was reminded again how lucky I had been to be able to take time out, to be in the position financially to do so. Other carers were not so lucky, I knew. As the train whisked me past old haunts, I re-read letters from those who had struggled to survive …

I spent nine years as a carer for my father. Being a carer in some ways honed me in steel and taught me the beauty of life, but it also showed me the ugly side. At the age of fifty-six I now live in a one-bedroom council flat. After Dad died, life on social security was not easy so I jumped in feet first and got a job as a cook and another as a cleaner. I am leaving the job as a cleaner as I go there straight from cooking and I am getting too tired. I would love to partake in some of life's pleasures now, but poverty does not allow for this.

(Maria, Newcastle)

After my father died I had a terrible time with social services. I wasn't entitled to any unemployment benefit because I had not worked for the last two years. I had inherited the house and so I wasn't entitled to any income support because I had too many 'savings'. I panicked because I had no income and didn't want to spend money knowing that I might have to sell my house to simply live. I had to get a job. I had no time to really take a break. And when I went to work as a van driver, I found that I was so exhausted that I couldn't work two straight days in a row. Just couldn't physically manage it. I could only work part-time and then was worried about money all over again.

(Peter, London)

After Mum died I had the most awful panic attacks but the DSS said I was fit to work and so I applied for a job at a local department store. To my horror I found that I just couldn't work one day straight after the other because I was completely exhausted. After all the years of pushing myself to work all hours as a carer it seemed my body was just refusing to allow that to happen again. Even working part-time I became very run-down and the doctor had to give me a certificate. It has been an awful struggle financially. I had just £49 a week to live on. I've been constantly caring. As a single Mum I brought up two children. And from age twenty-eight until almost fifty I cared for my parents. I feel strongly that all ex-carers should receive a pension in recognition of their work.

(Maggie, Cambridge)

I spent all my money that I had worked hard for over the years on improving the quality of life for my ill wife. I don't begrudge it. But now I am left living in poverty and with little or no help from the Government. I am of the age where finding work does not come easy. Life as a carer is hard. Life past caring is perhaps harder.

(Ian, Inverness)

As the cab draws up outside Ursula's house (a carer I had interviewed four years earlier*), her son Scott, now aged eleven and much taller, wider, growing into a fine young man, excitedly rushes down the path, gushing, "Would you like a cup of tea and a rich-tea biscuit?" He zooms off to the kitchen as I hug Ursula. She is now thirty-two years old. When we last met, Ursula had shared with me her dreams of getting an education. After seventeen years of caring, she had been about to begin college, studying for English and Maths GCSE. I want to know how her studies are going, how her dreams are shaping up. I want to know … everything.

---

* Ursula's first interview is on page 62

Ursula's Story (part 2)

I loved going to college. Learning gave me a sense of being alive, of truly living. It was scary but exciting. I learnt I could do things that I never knew I could. I surprised myself. Yes, there were days when I thought oh God, I can't do this, but Scott would help me with my homework, John too, they were very supportive. I enjoyed the social interaction. Us students were like a bag of liquorice all-sorts, a real mixture. I only went two days a week and it was tiring but in a good way. It hurt so much when I had to give up my studies.

Money. That was the problem. We couldn't survive on just the one wage. The debts, ever higher, were a terrible strain on John and me. We argue more now. He wanted me to work but even though I was only going to college two days a week, I couldn't work on the other days. I just didn't have the energy. In the end it was a case of food on the mind or food on the plate. I left college. I got a job back cleaning. I was angry, angry at myself, at John, at the State for not giving us enough support. My dreams, slashed. I was sore.

For over two years I worked as a private cleaner in a residential house. Then one day, I discovered a cyst on my breast. I was terrified. They cut it out. Thankfully it was benign. Recently I've been plagued by migraines. I used to hear people talk about migraines, that they hurt so. I used to think yeah, take a strong paracetemol, you'll be fine. Then it happened to me. Head exploding, splitting, paracetemol useless. I think it's like being a carer. It's not until it happens to you that you can really understand what its like.

I'm off work now with phlebitis. The doctor says I have to rest. I feel guilty because I know I can't afford to. But the doctor says the years of caring have left my immune system wrecked. I think I've been so ill because I had to dive right in so soon past caring and get a job. No chance for a breather. When you're caring you think oh, when the caring days are over I'll get on with my life, with college, family, whatever. The reality is different. Mentally you may wish to but physically you can't get on with anything. You don't know how worn out you are until you try to carry on and find you keep getting stopped.

This phlebitis is agony. I stay home. It gives me time with Scott. It gives me time with me, time in the mind. Five years on, I'm still grieving. Still miss Mum. Emotionally, physically, still battered, bruised.

One day I want to go back to college. I want to get my GCSEs. Get my certificate, have a photo of me, holding it up, I'm going to fight for that. I'm thirty-two now. I know that I still have many opportunities and possibilities before me. I may have lost the battle but not the war. I have to rest now but then I'm going to fight ... fight for my life.

* * *

Like a new-born babe gasping for breath, past carers are catapulted into a new world. Like a new-born babe they tire easily, need plenty sleep, food, nurture. They cry a lot. They need care and love to grow. In their quest for independence they discover their feet, shaky they topple, crawl, fall down and pull themselves up once more. They reach out to be supported, encouraged.

After the death of my parents, I took baby steps towards doing this book. I needed to raise money to fund the research, to go round the country interviewing past carers. I asked a friend, a businessman I had dated, if he might help me. His fortune was estimated at three hundred million pounds. I asked if he might be prepared to sponsor the research costs to the sum of £5,000. There would be a proper contract, money paid back (and hopefully more) when published. He said: "A book on caring? ... no, that'll never sell. Can't you think of something more commercial, more Jilly Cooper?"

Deflated, I temporarily gave up. I made up my mind that business people were cold and uncaring, only interested in profit.

Of course, had I really wanted to, I could have done the book, regardless. Problem was, I didn't believe in me. It wasn't the money I needed, but what it represented. The belief of someone else in me. I was stuck, stagnant without that. I hated myself for needing it. And, if not forthcoming, feeling even more helpless, I fought and defended, at war with the world.

My rich friend and I parted company. I knew – came to be aware – that my attraction to powerful men was because I so lacked power within myself. I saw that if I remained in such situations, I would become even more lacking. For ultimately, we cannot claim what belongs to another – and call it our own.

I decided I badly needed to find confidence. I went in search of it, as if it were something I might find on a supermarket shelf. I went to a homeopath and told her, "I'm looking for confidence." She laughed and said, "If I could bottle that I'd be a millionaire." I bought a Rough Guide and a backpack and set off on a long journey to Australia, Los Angeles, New York, searching. I swapped Henley for the New York Hudson, where a cat called Scotty and I lived on a blue-and-white rickety houseboat through two suffocating summers and a blue ice winter. A friend had given me a dilapidated laptop and I wrote about anything, everything. I wrote through the night, collapsing into bed as dawn showered the city pink. I chased super-confident American men whose pearl-white teeth gleamed as we kissed, me rubbing against them as if hoping their confidence might rub off on me, like glitter. (We remain creatures of habit even when we try not to be!) I drifted through this bright city as aimless as the dead body I once saw float down the Hudson. Through Central Park, in dark bars, on the self-help shelf in Barnes and Noble bookshops, confidence constantly sneaked away.

I grew tired. Weary.

I came home. I came home because there seemed no place left to go.

I bought a small flat a stones-throw from where I grew up, close to my brother Haig, my sister Fiona, a home where my wee nieces and nephews came with their laughter and fun, a home surrounded by a clan of cousins and aunts and uncles, my parents' brothers and sisters, who seemed to have lived here, in this tiny pocket of Edinburgh, forever.

I came home feeling a failure. Like something should have happened on my travels, I don't know what, just something. I had been all around the world looking for signs … where will I find a meaningful life? … and had ended up back where I had started.

So what now?

Half-heartedly I gathered some photos together and trekked round to a local acting agent. He looked at me and said: "But you were doing so well in London. What happened?"

One miserable rainy afternoon I settled down at home, a flat that overlooked the streets where I had skipped as a child. I thought, how the hell did I end up here? *What happened?* And what am I going to do? It seemed I had not done anything for so long and didn't know where to start even if I did know and oh I know, I know, yes, yes, perfect … I excitedly called my brother who I knew had been worried about me, in that protective way that older brothers are for their younger sisters, especially younger sisters who have no parents and seem to be drifting wild. I called him, thrilled I had come up with a plan, a master plan, why hadn't I thought of it before, it was perfect, now I had an answer, so many times he had said what are you going to do Audrey and so many times I had said I don't know and… "Hi Haig, listen, I know what I want to be … a grief counsellor!" Silence. "Isn't that great? I know that I could do that." He gave a little cough and said, "Audrey, don't you think you've seen enough suffering, been around enough dying and death? You're a young woman. What about life Audrey? What about *life?*"

That rainy afternoon I penned letters to various celebrities, strangers, telling them I was trying to do stories about life past caring and asking for their help. Imagine my delight when personally penned replies popped through my letterbox containing donations. Emma Thompson saying 'there is something so important about your project', Imogen Stubbs saying 'you have my total admiration, both my parents died when I was young and I was very lost'. Dame Judi Dench sending 'great good luck', Jane Asher offering sound practical advice, Natasha Richardson sending a card from New York, Matthew Kelly and his agent sending support, a card from a past carer, Doreen Davidson enclosing a donation with the words 'I think Fred would have liked you to have this', a donation on behalf of the Ambika Paul Charitable Foundation and one from a local businessman, Robbie Taylor from Taylor Castings, who had heard of the project and mentioned it to the director of Livingston Precision who sent something too. Then the Cross Trust gave me something and the Scottish Arts Trust.

Shock, horror! No more excuses. No more fighting, battling, saying the world is an awful place full of uncaring people. Suddenly people saying yes, we want to help, yes, we believe in the value of this book, yes, we believe you can do it, Audrey.

Oh No!

As I tentatively placed the advertisement asking for past carers to get in touch, I realised I had taken the first step on yet another journey, only this time I had no idea where it would lead me.

I fell down often, unsure of where to go next. I cried out for help. I discovered the healing touch of Reiki, the lightness of Osho Meditation, the inspiration of a course called The Landmark Forum. I bumped into old friends and new. In the summer of 2000 I sat with one of those friends, and we held hands as I blubbed non-stop for seven hours. We had met in town for 'a quick coffee'. It came without warning. There was nothing I could do to stop it. It happened *to* me. I couldn't care I was in a public place for the world seemed to disappear. I could hear my friend ordering more hot chocolate, cappuccino, camomile tea, yet I had no concept of time. All I knew was that my friend never once let go of my hand and afterwards took me home to her house, tucked me up in bed, made me dinner and later we watched a Tom Cruise video. And though I couldn't believe that I had howled for *seven* hours, and though I felt like I'd been run over by a steam-roller, we couldn't stop giggling as we realised the café staff would have thought we were breaking up (the café was in a gay part of town).

I came to understand that grief is like a river. Just when we think we are safely over it, we are once more swept away. Sometimes we are the swimmer, struggling. Sometimes it is as if we are standing on the bank, the surprised observer. The river flows at its own pace, mocking our attempts to make it go faster, slower. Life goes on. We go on, still. Deep below the surface, out of sight, things move, shift, rise. Sometimes there is the bursting of a dam. Sometimes there is merely a ripple. Healing happens with and without our knowing. The river knows best.

After seven years I climbed back on stage to discover my passion for acting had not died, but been merely anaesthetised. I stumbled into a man, an Irishman with a kind soul and a wicked wit, who did not run when I delivered my war cry 'don't get close, one day I'll be gone' but instead said, 'okay, okay, if that makes you happy. I just want you to be happy'. To my amazement I began to care again. I uncovered love. I recovered my roots and though two people less, there was my family. A brother, sister, nieces, nephews, in-laws, aunts, uncles, cousins, still there, a family I loved and to whom I belonged.

And as I searched for life, I met strangers along the way and we shared stories.

And almost without realising, the scenery slowly changed from black and white to colour.

For with the help of others, I came to understand that a meaningful life is whatever we choose to give meaning to.

It is ours to invent.

It is whatever we choose to care about, to be passionate about, whatever we would ache for and sweat for and speak up for and get out of bed for (provided, of course, this does not harm anyone else).

I learned that a meaningful life is everything and anything and nothing. For what matters is not the choice but that we are happy with the choice.

I came to see that my battle was not with the world, but with myself.

And I came to know that in being lost, we find.

> "We shall not cease from exploration
> And the end of all our exploring
> will be to arrive where we started
> And know the place for the first time."
> T. S. Eliot

Part 3

A RECOVERY GUIDE

A RECOVERY GUIDE

I'm worried about carers, about past carers. And so, based on what they've told me, I compiled a twelve-step recovery guide.

The steps are not in any particular order but can be done depending on how you feel that day. Don't worry if you feel you're not where you should be. I will never forget the words of a Hollywood screenwriter who, to the dismay of the studio bosses when asked how long it would take him to write a project, would say: "It takes as long as it takes."

I believe this is true of past caring. Recovery takes as long as it takes. We can only be where we are at. And so, wherever we are at is absolutely right for us. Life is, for the most part, a work in progress.

1. **Recovering a Sense of Being**

2. **Recovering a Sense of your own Health**

3. **Recovering a Sense of Peace**

4. **Recovering a Sense of Relationship**

5. **Recovering a Sense of Self-esteem**

6. **Recovering a Sense of Creativity**

7. **Recovering a Sense of Joy and Fun**

8. **Recovering a Sense of Sensuality**

9. **Recovering a Sense of Sexuality**

10. **Recovering a Sense of Purpose**

11. **Recovering a Sense of Possibility**

12. **Recovering a Sense of Strength**

Recovering a Sense of Being

allow yourself to stop, allow yourself to be ...

We live in a society where we move at such a frenetic pace and have so many demands on our time that no wonder we become disconnected from ourselves. Our feelings. Keeping busy is also a great way of avoiding what's really going on inside us.

Allow yourself to STOP

Don't feel bad, don't feel guilty about it. Others may try to stop you from stopping. They may try to keep you busy, tell you 'you must do *something*!' To do nothing goes against everything that our busy Western society tells us we must do in order to be happy. Get more money, a bigger house, a new car, fashionable clothes. In deciding to stop, you are saying hang on, my well-being – I – am more important than anything material. And this can be a threat to those busy people around us.

To make a deliberate decision to 'take time out' and do nothing is to do something very brave. It requires courage. Many people are too scared to stop because they fear they will get left behind. They fear being regarded by others as simply lazy or weak. Or they may fear the prospect of having to face their own feelings.

But recognising and owning how we feel is a major step towards healing and recovery of self.

EXERCISE

Lie down on the floor with a cushion under your head. If this is not comfortable, a bed will do, but take care to keep awareness. Cover yourself with a blanket. Make sure you are somewhere you won't be disturbed. Take three deep breaths, breathing in through the nose and exhaling through the mouth.

Acknowledge your body lying here covered with a blanket. Take a minute to really tune in to your body and your surroundings. Invite every muscle in your body to relax. Let the floor or bed take the full weight of your body, tell yourself that it is safe to let go, you are supported from your head to your toes. Work your way up … Wriggle your toes, tense them for five seconds and relax. Really let them flop. Now your ankles. Now calves, knees, upper leg, thighs, abdomen, chest, shoulders, back, arms, neck, face, scalp. Tense and relax.

Thank your body for all the incredible hard work it has done for you. Let it know that you truly appreciate that it has kept working for you in very difficult circumstances.

Apologise to your body for having neglected it for so long. Tell your body you are now here for it and you want to give it the best care and attention.

Now gently ask your body to let you know how it feels. Sensations may come up in the form of physical pain. Or perhaps emotions. If nothing comes up, don't worry. Just keep gently asking your body, inviting it to let you know how it feels right now.

Keep breathing gently, without force.

Listen. What is your body trying to tell you? If an emotion arises don't stifle it, just allow yourself to be with it. There is no-one else to see, you are safe. It may feel uncomfortable but just try to keep with it, let it happen.

Ask your body gently, what can I do for you? What can I do to help you? Listen. What is your body telling you it needs?

For example:
If your body tells you it needs to sleep, sleep.
If your body tells you it needs to cry, cry.
If your body tells you there is an ache, listen to where it aches.

If your body doesn't know what it wants right now acknowledge that is okay not to know, you understand it needs space to discover how it feels and that you will be there to help it when it is ready.

Allow yourself at least twenty minutes to stop. Tune in to the breath, keep the jaw relaxed. A good way to re-energise is to imagine that you are breathing in positive energy on the in-breath and breathing out negative energy on the out-breath. You may like to imagine the positive energy as warm and a colour; a vibrant colour like silver or gold, flowing like a warm river through the body. Imagine this positive energy is reaching every cell, every organ. Imagine the heavy, tired energy is dissolving out through the skin as the positive energy replaces it.

Always end the exercise by thanking your body for letting you know how it feels. Assure your body that you now have the time again to devote to it and that you will be listening out for it on a daily basis.

Stop … listen … feel …

Recovering a Sense of your own Health

Caring for ... You

In caring for someone else our own health suffers.

Worry, stress and anxiety affects our appetites, makes us feel more like 'nourishing' our bodies with endless cups of tea, coffee, cigarettes, and sugary things like chocolate and cakes. These substances give us instant energy but we feel more tired and 'down' soon afterwards. So we need more stimulants to keep us going. And so on.

Every single day our bodies require adequate vitamins and minerals to repair daily cellular damage and keep internal organs in good working order. Stress is known to affect the efficiency of the immune system – it is well-known that stressed-out souls are more prone to cold, flu and all sorts of infections.

> Eating well is quite simply one of the most
> important things you can do.

Caring is a major drain on the body's physical and emotional resources. It may seem a real effort to cook for yourself but it is worth it. Not only will you feel more able to cope physically but also mentally. Have you ever noticed how much better you feel after a healthy meal than a stodgy plate of grease? This is because food affects our moods and emotions.

So next time you think, oh, what's the point of cooking, it's only me, I'll just have toast ... Stop ... think again ... You matter. Your body matters.

If you live alone and are finding the days and weeks immediately past caring too tough to think about shopping, making a meal or doing anything domestic (some carers report they can hardly wash or dress themselves) perhaps you have some dear friends you could stay with for a week or so? (Not for too long though as this may result in becoming quite dependent on them.)

You may have been invited to stay with friends and feel guilty about being a burden or being in the way. But if your friends or relatives are truly there, ready to care for you, then why not?

Past carers are undoubtedly run-down emotionally, physically, mentally and spiritually and deserve a little pampering to help them in their recovery.

So if the offer is there, enjoy it for a while.

Long-term, though, we are responsible for our health and looking after ourselves.

Recovering a Sense of Peace

Forgiving yourself

Forgiveness is a major step to self-healing. We never get it absolutely right. There is no neat manual, no life 'how-to' guide.

Carers cannot control another person's illness or what is going to happen that day. Nobody can, not the best doctors or even the person who is ill. The natural cycle of dying is bigger than us. And so we have to stumble through in the dark. Sometimes we'll feel overwhelmed, unsure, terrified. Sometimes we'll act or react in ways we later regret.

Past caring, we may feel tremendous guilt about what we did or didn't do. But carers are only human and humans make mistakes. We learn by our mistakes. How can we know about the best way to deal with a situation until we have lived through it? If we had known then what we know now we might have handled it differently. But, like any new experience we learn only by living it.

Be gentle, be easy on yourself.

Forgive yourself for all the things that you said or didn't say.

Forgive yourself for the one thing that you forgot to do in the hundred, thousands you did.

Forgive yourself for not knowing what to do, for only knowing *after* the event.

Forgive yourself. At the time you did your best.
This is all we can do.

This is all we can ever do.

EXERCISE

Sit or lie down in a comfortable position and cover yourself with a blanket. Make sure you will not be disturbed.

Take three deep breaths, inhaling through the nose and out through the mouth. As you exhale allow the jaw to relax and let go of any tension in the throat.

Cup your hands about an inch from your throat and imagine that a warm circle of golden light is shining from your hands right onto your Adam's Apple. Imagine the warm golden light gently soaking through your pores and opening up your throat, releasing any tension there, allowing your voice-box to be relaxed and free.

Remember to breathe deeply but gently, without force.

During this exercise you may find that specific images or memories come up. You may feel physical sensations or emotions. Just allow these feelings to be there, acknowledge them, be aware of them, all the time gently repeating the affirmation.

If it feels too uncomfortable, then stop and just breathe gently. Try to stay with the feelings you are experiencing. Breathe gently until you feel you are able to continue the exercise.

Now on a soft out-breath say out loud the following statements:

    I forgive myself for all the things I didn't know

    I forgive myself for all the things I couldn't know

    I forgive myself for all the things I didn't, couldn't know

And on a soft out-breath:

    I forgive myself for all the things I didn't say

    I forgive myself for all the things I couldn't say

    I forgive myself for all the things I didn't, couldn't say.

You can choose to make up your own affirmations that may be particularly helpful to you. Start your sentence with 'I forgive myself for …' and add in whatever is appropriate for you. I find it is helpful to repeat the same affirmation three times.

A good way to end the exercise is by saying out loud …

I (and here you can insert your name) accept I did my best in the circumstances.

You may find it helpful to write a letter to your loved one. This exercise can help with clearing what was left unsaid. Writing things down in the form of a letter may help you to understand your own feelings better too.

Another useful exercise is to imagine the person in front of you and you can tell them how you feel. You may like to do this alone or ask an understanding friend to play the part of your loved one. Allow any emotions to come up, knowing that you are safe.

You may find it helpful to seek professional help, such as working with a trained counsellor, to help resolve feelings of guilt or unforgiveness towards yourself or others.

Forgiving ourselves is a vital part of the recovery process.

Recovering a Sense of Relationship

Friends, lovers, strangers, relations

Re-building a sense of relationship with others is a step towards re-building a 'social' life. A life of sharing a part of yourself, emotionally or physically, with others.

It may feel strange and uncomfortable to open up and let others become a regular part of your life. Acknowledge that fear. It is natural after a long time of being socially isolated.

If you call an old friend you haven't spoken to in a long time and feel nervous, then you may like to begin by saying ... hi, I feel a little nervous about calling you after such a long time, but I've been thinking about you recently and wondering what you were up to ... I'd really like to catch up ...

You may be lucky to have friends that, no matter how long goes by, you easily take up from where you left off. Why not call one of those friends now and arrange to meet for coffee? Or a night out? Don't be afraid to make the first move but ...

Be prepared ... that your friend's life will have moved on and they may be busy doing things that you may have wished for but were not able to do. Perhaps they have been travelling or got married or had a child. Accept that your life has followed a different path but now you may be in a position to do all those things you couldn't when you had caring responsibilities. Rather than feeling jealous or bitter, see this as an opportunity to hear all about your friend's experiences, knowing that you, too, will perhaps now be able to develop those areas of your life that have so far been neglected. See it as a way of learning, of gleaning knowledge. For example, if your friend has travelled, and you want to do that in the future, get tips, information. Quiz them. How was it? Where were the best places? What was the food like, the weather?

Be prepared … that some 'friends' will not know what to say to you. Many people don't know how to react to death. It is unfortunately a subject that our society tends to shy away from. It could be that you wish to talk about what you've been through and your friend keeps changing the subject. The truth is they may not know what to say. Unless their situation has been similar, they will have no idea what it feels like to have gone through what you have. You may feel hurt, angry at his or her apparently uncaring attitude. So make it easier for you and them. If you are needing to talk about your grief, call a recognised counsellor or your local carers' organisation who will be able to put you in touch with the right person. Sometimes it is actually easier to talk to a stranger. They will listen impartially, without judgement, and anything you say will be in total confidence.

Be prepared … that you may meet your friend and find that you really have nothing in common any more. (This does not just happen if you have been a carer). Don't feel bad. Accept that people move in different directions and through their experiences see the world differently. This is simply part of the process of life … friends come in many shapes and forms, some are close to us at certain points in our life then drift away, some friends may be there with us to the grave. If you feel it's no longer a true friendship, acknowledge and appreciate the friendship you did once share with that person, remember the good times. And gently let go.

LOVERS

When caring perhaps you found it impossible to establish any kind of romantic relationship. Or perhaps a relationship broke up because of caring demands? Maybe you were caring for your spouse and it was difficult to maintain any kind of physical intimacy? (I talk about sex and sensuality in another recovery chapter. But let's for the moment concentrate on how to recover a social life).

You may feel rather daunted at the idea of dating again. But meeting new people can be fun. We all have different life experiences to share and there are new experiences in the future to share together too.

If you have not had a relationship for many years because you have been caring, and you feel nervous about sharing that with a potential partner, don't panic and make up some story. Simply tell the truth. If the person is worth anything, they will respect what you have done. They might not understand it but they will respect it. If they don't, they're not worth it. They're not worth *you*.

People can meet in any situation at any moment ... At bus-stops, in cafés, on the tube, in a club or bar.

Through mutual friends, dating agencies, classified ads – whether by placing one yourself or answering one. (Note: if you are meeting someone through a dating agency, a newspaper ad or through the internet, *always* meet in a mutual place and tell someone where you are going. Carry a mobile phone if possible and never give out your home address until you feel absolutely comfortable with the person.)

Take up a new hobby, sport; join a gym, do voluntary work, sign up for a singles holiday, attend a past carers support group, other support group or a night-class to learn a new skill.

We have no control over who we meet and if we will 'click' with them. What we do have control over is the ability to widen our social circle. It just requires a little bit of courage – but then you already have loads of that – otherwise how could you have cared?

RELATIVES

There may be members of our family who we are not talking to, with whom we fell out. Perhaps the stress of the caring situation caused a breakdown in relations? How do you feel about this now? Do you miss them? You may wish to seek counselling about this and the best way to deal with your feelings around this issue.

If you feel you would like to re-establish relations with estranged loved ones, why not start by writing them a letter? You may prefer to telephone but if there is a lot to say a letter is often better. You have a space to say what you want without being interrupted and risk the conversation going way off at a tangent. You can explain what you felt then and what you feel now. Tell them that you would like to see them again. (Remember we have no control over the person's response, the only thing we have control over is our own actions).

Perhaps you feel bitter or angry toward members of your family about the way you were treated – or the way they treated the person you were caring for? Those feelings are common. You are not odd or strange to feel them. You should seek counselling for this as feelings of unresolved anger often turn into depression. Contact your local carers' centre, they should be able to put you in touch with someone who can help. Counsellors are specially trained and will help you to find a way to resolve these issues depending on your circumstances.

Perhaps there was not a fall out, but you simply lost touch with some family members in much the same way that you lost touch with your friends? Caring meant there was no time to socialise or visit. Why not visit relatives you've lost touch with now, or invite them to visit you? Make a day of it. Arrange to meet for lunch or coffee. Take some photos of your loved one along and share some memories. Laugh and cry together. I am still amazed when I meet up with my aunts and they tell me things about my Mum and Dad, things that they did when they were children or other things about my family that I had no idea about. It tickles me to hear these stories, and adds to my bigger picture of my parents' lives before I popped along.

Recovering a social life check list:

Sharing yourself with others in honesty and truth.

Enjoying a new hobby or sport.

Doing some voluntary work, something you care about but that's also fun for you.

Ringing up old friends, new friends.

Being part of a group, a support group or some other group that stands for something you believe in.

Seeking help when you need it.

Mending old family quarrels for no other reason than you want to.

Sharing memories and laughing.

Relating to others, valuing yourself and others.

Having a social life!

Recovering a Sense of Self-esteem

Pamper yourself
Not luxury, necessity

> All my life I have been caring for others. I now find the biggest challenge is to care for me.
>
> *(Margaret, 56, a carer for twenty-five years)*

Please ... don't feel guilty about being good to yourself. When we embark on recovering a sense of our own worth we need to treat ourselves with extra TLC (tender loving care).

Out of necessity, someone else's needs came first. We neglected our own needs. Now we must learn how to tune in, listen and respond to our needs again.

You may feel confused about what your needs are. This is natural. When we are pouring our energy into the well-being of someone else, the little voice inside that cries 'what about me?' gets ignored. This little voice grows tired and fainter until it finally gives up. It decides it didn't matter anyway.

Tuning-in again to that little voice can feel odd when we are not used to it. We may try to smother it, thinking, it's silly to do something nice just for me ... that's selfish, isn't it? ... others matter more ... I'm not worth bothering about ... I only want to help others.

We can only truly help others when we have a healthy attitude towards helping ourselves. Sometimes we have to be a little selfish, to give ourselves time and space before we embark on helping others. Forever helping others can be a way of avoiding ourselves, our own lives.

Recovering self-esteem means we can choose to help others in a healthy way.

Only when we support and nurture ourselves are we truly able to support and nurture others.

The world puts the same value on you that you put on yourself. Recovering self-esteem involves treating yourself well, with respect, with love. It is about learning to say 'no' when you really don't want to do something. It is about surrounding yourself with loving people who treat you well, who value you. Avoid people who drag you down, who constantly criticise, nag or are angry with you. (When you learn to really value yourself these sorts of people soon drop out of your life automatically. Those who try to dominate others are usually lacking self-esteem themselves and tend to attract those with even less self-esteem).

Hanging onto a sense of self-esteem whilst in the company of others can sometimes prove difficult. Humans tend to compare themselves with each other. This is a torturous trap. There will always be someone else more pretty, more handsome, slimmer, popular, more wealthy, more successful, more …

It is wise to only compare ourselves with ourselves. To ask, how am I doing now compared with how I was doing a year ago?

Recovering self-esteem involves doing things for ourselves that help us feel good about ourselves. It is important to find what works for you but below are some suggestions.

The Bath

Put towels on a radiator or to heat by a fireplace.

Run yourself a deep warm bath, you may like to add a couple of drops of your favourite essential oil. Lavender and camomile are good ones to aid relaxation. You could play soft, soothing music. Light a scented candle. Soak in the bath. Breathe deeply. If the phone rings, don't answer it. If you have children, tell them not to disturb you. Savour the sensation of warm water on your skin, the vibration of the music, the aroma of the candle. Savour the fact that you have created this just for you. If you begin to feel guilty remind yourself that if you are to feel better you must start to value yourself and that means treating yourself well.

Close your eyes.

Imagine that all your worries are melting through the pores of your skin and into the bath water.

Breathe deeply.

Soak for about twenty minutes (bearing in mind that any longer may have an overly-drying effect on the skin).

As you climb out of the bath, wrap yourself in the heated towels. Imagine your worries are disappearing down the plughole.

Dry yourself off and smooth on your favourite body lotion (for men too!) (Cocoa butter smells wonderful!)

Put on your dressing gown; wrap yourself in a blanket or duvet and lie down on the sofa or in bed. Give yourself an hour. Do whatever you want. If you want to read, read. Nap. Daydream. Write. Relax. Whatever. You are creating this for you.

When you get up you could perhaps make yourself a cup of revitalising tea. Dress in your favourite colours, put on a little make-up or jewellery or a colourful scarf or special cuff links or those soft woollen socks. For no other reason than you choose to.

If you have your bath in the evening, make yourself a cup of relaxing tea such as camomile or Roobois (tea with no caffeine but tastes just like a real cuppa.) Cosy in and have an early night. Do this weekly, if not more.

Treat Yourself

Once a week buy yourself a little present. It doesn't have to be expensive. Just a few pounds. How about a second-hand book or CD, or a bunch of flowers, a new toothbrush, a punnet of strawberries, a crystal, an inspirational card. A bag full of your favourite sweets. A plant. A special pen. A new kind of cheese. A candle. A funny key ring. Seeds for a window-box.

Tune Into Yourself ...

You could try ...

    a meditation group
    a relaxation group
    a gentle yoga class
    a reiki session

Many of the larger cities have reiki sessions available by donation only. Some meditation classes are free or by donation. Any reputable health food store or alternative therapy centre may have details.

Many past carers I spoke to used their local library as a resource centre. Sometimes it was simply a warm place to go to get out of the house. You can browse through the papers, read your favourite books or surf the net. You may see something that you would like to try or that gives you a new idea. Remember you are looking for ways to nurture yourself.

If you have a bit more money to spend, how about treating yourself to a massage, a manicure, a pedicure, that new haircut or outfit? What about having your colours done by a professional? Or how about making a day trip or a weekend away to see friends, or booking a holiday to somewhere you've always dreamed of going?

Keep a diary of what you did for yourself each day/week and of how you felt afterwards.

Make a 'wish list' of ten things you would like to do for yourself. Tick them off as you do them.

List ten qualities you like about yourself. Really show off. Go on!

Learn to say 'No' – and 'Yes'!

Be as good to yourself as you would a dear friend.

Value yourself ... and others will too.

Recovering a Sense of Creativity

A creative recovery is a healing process
Creativity is therapy and therapy is creativity.

> I write poetry and that helped me. I've a few poems published, but y'know, it doesn't matter if they were never published, the reward would be the same. I think if you're passionate about something, whether it looks good to someone else or not, isn't the point. The point is that it provides a creative outlet for you, brings you to a greater understanding of yourself. If someone else happens to like it too, then that's a bonus. Others may want to constantly criticise you, hinder you. Try to avoid them, life's too short. Try to surround yourself with loving people, who wish to nurture you.
>
> *(Margaret, a carer for her husband David)*

You may feel like you are the sort of person who could never be creative. But the truth is, we all, each and every one, have the ability to be creative in some way. We are creative without even realising it. Choosing what colours to decorate our homes in is a creative act. Deciding how to arrange the furniture, where to hang paintings, even how to arrange the food on our plates all requires a degree of creativity.

Creativity is in abundance in the universe. A walk in nature can be special, so uplifting, as we witness the perfection of nature at work. Without force, a flower opens. A river flows. Night turns into day. Water on a leaf evaporates and the roots immediately circulate more water to the leaf. Birds sing. Clouds burst. We are surrounded by so much creative energy, no wonder some of it rubs off on us without our realising!

At the moment you may feel you are too dead inside to be creative. This is normal after a trauma.

I bumped into Louise. We had been friends at school and had not seen each other in years. The last I heard she had graduated from art school and was a dedicated painter. I was surprised to see her working as an Arts administrator. She told me that, since her father's death two years before, she had not been able to pick up a paintbrush.

One Christmas, browsing in a bookshop, I suddenly found myself beside Calum, my old acting professor at Drama School. His intense passion and commitment to the craft of acting and the theatre had inspired many a fledgling Olivier and Leigh. I asked if he had seen any good plays recently. He said he hadn't set foot inside a theatre in three years. He couldn't bear to. Not since he had watched his sister die of cancer.

Loss kills passion. You may feel that the passion you once had for a person or a creative activity has died. But creative energy, if used positively, can be healing.

It can also be destructive. It is important to channel the energy in a way that gives you power.

Construct … don't destruct …

EXERCISE

Make a list of any creative activity that you once enjoyed before you became a carer. Without forcing, gently ask yourself how you feel about trying these activities now? If nothing inspires you, or if you never considered yourself creative before, then how about trying something new? Just gently plant a few seeds. You may find it useful to join a local class in your chosen activity. This could also open up your social life and allow you to be supported by others.

Creativity is a form of expression ... self-expression.

Some suggestions ... add your own too

Dancing

Dance in a class or dance alone in the safety of your house.

Writing

Join a writing class where you share your work, or keep a private diary. After the death of his parents, Dave Eggers at the age of twenty-one inherited his little brother, age seven. He went to creative writing classes in California and later wrote a novel about his experiences called *A Heartbreaking Work of Staggering Genius*. It became a best-seller.

Sculpture

The notorious Glasgow hard man Jimmy Boyle found a way to express his inner self through sculpture and saved himself from a continuing life of crime.

Reading Groups

Most local libraries have a reading group that meet monthly and discuss a book. Conversation, debate, can be creative. Many books, from poetry to prose, have been inspired from broken hearts.

Painting

Join a painting or drawing class or what about a night-school course studying the great Masters? The Mexican painter Frida Kahlo painted whilst bedridden after a serious road accident at the age of fifteen destroyed her dreams of being a doctor.

Cooking

What about collecting favourite recipes and adding some of your very own to make a little booklet? You could decorate it with a design and give them to friends. Nigella Lawson famously gave up journalism for cooking after her husband became ill with cancer so she could spend more time at home.

Redecorate the house

Experiment. Be daring. Use colours that you would never have before!

Sewing/knitting/dress-making

Make yourself a skirt, a top, a hair-band. Stella McCartney designed for and headed an anti-fur campaign that also reflected the beliefs of her mother Linda, who died from breast cancer.

Pottery

Take up a pottery class and make yourself a present!

Keep Fit

Join a gym and beat hell out of the punchbag! Not only great for getting fit but for letting off steam.

Adventure

Ever fancied putting on a back-pack and taking off to some far-flung place? Jonny Gibb, the winner of ITV's *Survivor,* put his travelling plans on hold when he was eighteen to help care for his sisters (then aged eight and thirteen), after his Mum died of skin cancer. Jonny and a friend, John Dalzell, set out to tackle Mount Kilimanjaro in Tanzania and helped raise more than £20,000 for Macmillan Cancer Relief in memory of his mother.

Music/Singing
What about joining a choir? Or learning to play a musical instrument?

Acting
Ever fancied treading the boards? Or helping backstage? Is there a local amateur dramatic society in your area? Emma Thompson's father suffered a stroke when she was a budding actress. She went on to win an Oscar.

We all, each and every one have a creative centre.

Avoid people who only want to criticise. Seek out people who are creative and nurturing, who encourage you in your creative activities and healing. And don't criticise yourself. We were all beginners at the beginning! Be generous with yourself.

Nurturing our creativity involves nurturing ourselves.

Recovering a sense of Joy and Fun

What's that again?
Stress makes you feel like you've had the stuffing kicked out of
you! It drains our life-force and drives joy into hiding.

Caring for someone we love, watching them slowly die, our spirit dies a little too. Joy and fun take a long holiday and you may believe, right now, that they will never return. It may seem they have been missing for months. Years. Perhaps you have forgotten the sound of your own laughter?

Laugh now. Just gently laugh for no other reason than to listen to the sound. Just a soft laugh, just to hear the basic sound. It may sound thin, false, insincere. But the basic sound is still there.

The truth is that joy and fun never leave us completely. Joy and fun live within us always, but sometimes they go to sleep, hibernate for many years, until it is safe to return.

When you feel that you may never know joy again, that everything is pointless and meaningless, acknowledge that this is a healthy, natural response to the trauma you have been through. Let your spirit know that you understand how it feels and that you are there to help it to recover those feelings when it feels ready.

You may feel you will never know joy and fun but I bet there was a time in your life when you did know them well ...

EXERCISE

Cover yourself with a blanket, make sure you will not be disturbed. Close your eyes. Breathe deeply and slowly three times, imagining you are breathing in positive energy from the air and breathing out any negativity.

Now gently invite yourself to go on a journey. Invite yourself to remember a time in your life when you felt the sensation of joy. For the purpose of the exercise it is best to remember a time when you were alone feeling joyful. It may have been a long time ago, way back before your caring days. It may have been when you were a child. It may have been a time when you were caring. It may have been related to a specific event or for no reason except it was one of those beautiful sunny days when it felt good to be alive.

Remember the sensation of lightness and a spring in your step. Recall that lovely warm feeling of being relaxed, at ease, feeling at one with the world. What were you doing? Perhaps you were reading a good book curled by the fire, or walking through the park, or watching children playing or cooking or enjoying a hobby, making something for yourself. Perhaps you are watching a funny film on telly or listening to the radio or dancing around the house on your own to your favourite song.

Remember to breathe … let any images, memories surface. If nothing comes, don't worry, the time is not ready yet. Just keep relaxing and inviting the memory and sensations of joy to surface. Recovery takes time and the body knows best.

If images of joy arise, be with the memory and be aware of how it feels in the body now, lying here, as you recall those images. You don't have to do anything with it, except be aware of it.

Now slowly open your eyes. Take a few moments to become fully present to your surroundings. Wriggle your hands and toes, become fully present to where you are now.

You may wish to write down any images that came to you. Perhaps there was something you were doing or a place that came up in your memory of joy. If you can, why not make a point of doing that thing again in your life now. Just try it out, with no expectations. Experiment. Certainly don't force it if you don't feel like it. Go for a walk along that beach or put the radio on and dance like a mad thing. Or rent a funny video. Whatever you choose. Don't worry if you don't feel any joy this time, just be with whatever emotion comes up, this is right for you at this point in life. And perhaps remembering something you once enjoyed doing will help you feel a little better today?

Recovering Fun

In Julia Cameron's *The Artist's Way*, the author suggests one day a week to be designated as a Play-date. The only condition is that you spend the day on your own and do something fun. You basically take yourself out for the day. I think this is a lovely idea.

If the whole day on your own seems a bit much, then why not arrange to spend the morning on your own and then meet a friend in the afternoon and do something together? I would recommend though, for the purpose of this exercise, that you don't just meet and chat. Make a point of actually *doing* something together, a specific action or outing.

Or you may want to spend the morning on your own and then join a group activity or class for the afternoon?

If you are feeling utterly exhausted or if the idea of being out of the house on your own is a bit scary, then how about taking yourself out just for an hour or two? Not far from home so you can get back easily should you need to.

Whatever you choose to do, try to ensure it may be *fun*! Try to choose something that takes you out of your normal routine. No voluntary work and *nothing* to do with caring, please!

I've listed some ideas you could do on your own or with a friend (some of which will depend on your own area and what they offer.) Why not add your own too?

A visit to a photographic exhibition or art gallery.

A barefoot walk along the beach and a paddle if warm enough!

Browsing round a bookshop/antique shop, just taking loads of time to potter.

Going to listen to some lunchtime music.

A gentle exercise class/yoga/dance class.

A walk round botanical gardens or a beautiful park.

A bus trip down the coast or to explore another part of town.

A visit to the museum.

Going swimming.

Going to that nice café in town for a creamy hot chocolate.

A trip round the charity shops.

A trip round that posh department store.

Taking up a painting or pottery class.

A horse-back riding lesson.

Taking a boat trip.

Joining a book group at your local library.

Learning a new language.

Going ice-skating.

Visiting a special church or cathedral.

Taking a city bus tour.

Going for a cycle ride.

Going to the cinema (complete with ice-cream and popcorn).

A visit to a Paint-your-own-Pottery shop (again, bigger cities have those shops, great for making wee gifts and excellent therapy).

A walk in the hills.

A visit to an animal rescue centre.

A game of ten-pin bowling or tennis or badminton or snooker.

Learning to drive (though that may be more stressful than fun!)

A class in how to make jewellery.

Having your make-up done professionally (a lot of the larger stores do this for no or a small charge).

A visit to a sea-bird centre, nature reserve or local place of interest.

Join a Biodanza class. Great fun and wonderful for integrating mind and body.

Recovering a Sense of Sensuality

Sight sound taste smell touch
Recovering our senses …

When we are under stress the world may feel heightened or deadened. We may be more acutely aware of our five senses; sight, sound, taste, smell and touch. Or we may feel numb to them.

Recovering a sense of sensuality is about recovering a sense of balance and harmony in the way that we interact with the world.

When we are under stress our nervous system is on the alert, pumping adrenaline ready for flight or fight. Our nerves are on edge, jangling. We can no longer bear the noise of the traffic, the sound of laughing, even the sound of people talking. It feels like we are experiencing sensory overload.

Imagine how the sound of a cup smashing on the floor sounds when you are stressed compared to when you are calm. If we are tense, the slightest unexpected sound or touch can startle us.

The body has its own way of coping with this. It can shut down the senses. It detaches you from them. This is what people mean when they describe 'looking at the world through a veil'.

When we are in good heart, we appreciate our surroundings. We hear the birdsong, we smell the freshly cut grass, we feel the sensation of a lover's touch on our skin.

When we are out-of-sorts we do not notice much. Or we notice too much!

Recovering a sense of sensuality brings us back in touch with our self and the world. To be sensitive is to be alive.

You can begin to recover your sensuality by doing things *consciously*, by shutting out all other distractions and focusing in on one sensory experience. Have you ever noticed how many of us use music as a background noise instead of really listening to it? Same with the television. It is often used as a familiar back-drop whilst we try to have a conversation or do something else. Little wonder our senses get overloaded.

Below are some exercises you could try. Remember, they are only suggestions.

Sound
Make a cuppa, put your feet up and listen to your favourite piece of music.

Touch
Feel the texture of a tree bark, a silk scarf, a rose petal. Close your eyes. How do they feel now?

Taste
Make a conscious decision to chew your food at least twenty times before swallowing. Taste every bit of it. Don't watch telly, don't talk to someone else. Just taste ... every single mouthful.

Smell
Buy three small scented candles and place them around the house. Compare them. Which one is your favourite? Why? How does it make you feel?

Sight
Go for a walk for no other reason than to observe. How many shades of colour make up the sky? What colour are the shops painted? What are people wearing? How do they look?

If you live near the sea or a pond dip your toe or hand in the water. What's the temperature like? What are the smells of the sea, the pond? Can you smell the seaweed? Close your eyes. Listen to the waves, the ripples. Touch the rocks, the sand, the stones. Can you hear the birds? What's the weather like? How does the rain feel? The sun? The wind? Treat yourself to an ice-cream or chips or whatever you fancy. Close your eyes. Smell the food. What does it remind you of, if anything? Taste the food. Savour it. Eat slowly.

Walk slowly. Talk slowly. Do everything slowly, with awareness.

Touch your own bare skin. How does it feel? Soft? Dry? Touch different parts of your body, the parts we often forget about, the backs of the knee, the tips of the fingers, the inner arm. Massage yourself gently around your belly button in a clockwise direction. How does it feel? (you may want to use a little almond oil). Close your eyes. Let your hand glide around your skin, exploring.

If you have a partner you may like to involve them in this exercise. After exploring your own body, gently explore your partner's skin. How does it feel?

Gently nourishing our senses every day

Recovering a Sense of Sexuality

Caring isn't sexy. It's messy, not sexy

Caring can make us feel asexual. We often lose touch with our sexual energy, with our sense of masculinity, femininity.

> Three months after my husband died I spied an advert in the paper for a makeover. A woman came to my house and basically went through my entire wardrobe … and threw away half my clothes! She told me I was dressing much too old for my years. I went out and bought some new clothes. I pampered myself. I treated myself to a facial and got my eyebrows waxed. I signed up for body-balance and jive classes. I felt like I was on a mission to re-invent myself.
>
> *(Martha, 52, a carer for her husband, John)*

In times of stress, sex goes out the window. We give up on it. Or we learn that it is not possible at that time and we learn to bury, repress our desire.

In recovering a sense of our sexual self we become aware of ourselves again as men and women, we become aware of our bodies and the fact that they can give us, indeed are designed, for sexual pleasure. We take care of our bodies and our minds so that when we do want to have sex it will be a joy rather than a pain, either emotionally or physically.

Study your body in a full-length mirror. Whenever we look at ourselves we have an immediate tendency to criticise. We're too fat, too thin, too something or other … but how about our good points? Our eyes, our neck, our hair, the colour of our skin? Compliment yourself. Become a friend of your body. Now gently ask yourself, is there anything that you could do that would make your body look and feel better? Have you had the same hair-style for years? Do you always wear the same dull colours? How about something brighter? Try different colours against your skin tone and see what happens. Some colours drain us, others make us look ten years younger. What about make-up? Is it years since you wore lipstick? How about treating yourself? Men, is it time to shave off the beard, the moustache? Admire yourself from all angles, looking not for faults but how you may take care of yourself in a way that will add to your feeling of attractiveness. Remember you're doing this for you, not anybody else!

Even if you do not have a partner there are plenty of steps you can take to get back in touch with your sexual being. You may feel embarrassed but sexual energy is a natural, healthy part of being alive. Even though our society can try to make it otherwise, it is certainly nothing to be ashamed of.

If you have not had sex for a long time, chances are you will be feeling insecure about having sex again. Sex is an area where almost everybody feels insecure, fears rejection or 'not being good enough'. We may feel afraid to say what we like, what we don't like, what we would like to try. We fear looking silly.

Before we attempt to give pleasure to another, it may be a good idea to get to know our own body again. When caring, or going through any trauma, our bodies and emotions often go numb. Start by gently awakening your sexual centre.

The following are some ideas and suggestions that may be helpful. (Have fun inventing some of your own too!)

Consciously become a friend again of your vagina or penis. Soak in a long hot bath. Dry and lie naked on the bed. Lock the door, unplug the phone, close the curtains, make sure the children are elsewhere and get to know your body. You may find it useful to use a hand-mirror. Study shape and form and explore with your fingers. What feels good? What feels not so good?

You may like to masturbate. Remember if guilty thoughts arise this is most likely a result of our 'conditioning' in society. It is perfectly natural to masturbate at any age.

You may like to experiment with a vibrator or a sex aid. These are easily purchased in the chain store Ann Summers and are also available through mail order. Again, if you feel embarrassed, be reassured that a broad spectrum of humanity can be found in those shops browsing … and buying.

Give yourself space to get back in touch with yourself.

If you have a partner or someone you have met and are planning to have a sexual relationship with, invite them to share with you some of the recovery exercises. If you are insecure about having sex, explain that you feel nervous because it has been a long time and you need to take things slowly.

So often sex is something squeezed into a busy life. It is often left until late at night when we are our most exhausted after a long day.

So why not plan it for an afternoon, an early evening? Clean the house, buy some sweet-smelling roses, put on fresh sheets. (Even if you are exploring your sexuality on your own it helps to create a 'sacred space' to do so in.)

You may want to begin by having a bath together and giving each other a light massage afterwards. Put on some soothing music, light scented candles, create a cosy, magical ambience.

Start with a long, long hug, lie in each other's arms listening to the music, tickle, stroke, kiss each other's bodies. Give yourselves plenty of time, no rushing. Don't have any telly on in the background or any other distractions. Be honest and open with one another. Give each other encouraging feedback. Ask your partner, how does that feel? If something doesn't feel good, softly whisper, actually that feels really good right there. You can help by moving their hand to the area, showing them what you mean or changing position.

If you trust and feel at ease with your lover, you may like to try the following exercise to awaken the sexual senses. One person lies down with a silk scarf tied very lightly over their eyes. The other person has a few minutes to go round the house and find ten objects to do with the senses smell, touch, sound and taste. It could be the smell of coffee, or an essential oil or the taste of ice-cream or the feel of a comb being run over the skin or a furry glove or the sound of a bell or a piece of music or … have fun with it. Use the parts of the body often neglected but that are teeming with nerve endings, the inner flesh of the lower arm, the back of the knees, the feet … the other person has to guess what the object is. Then swap over and do the same thing.

Past caring, I cut off emotionally from my body. Just numbed out. I've found the study and practise of Tantric sex very useful in bringing my entire being into the sex act. The idea of Tantric sex is that the sex act does not become about 'performance' but rather entering a meditative state where the mind lets go, relaxes, empties. Sex and love becomes about connecting to not only others but ourselves in the deepest place of our being.

There are numerous books available on the art of Tantric . It can be done as a couple or alone.

One lazy afternoon read *The Vagina Monologues* – men will get as much from it as women. Or *The Joy of Sex*. Or Nancy Friday. Anything that gets you back in touch with your sexual centre.

Recovering a Sense of Purpose

What gives our life meaning?

One of the hardest things to come to terms with is loss of purpose in life.

At the moment it may feel that nothing will ever give us such a strong sense of purpose again. What could be more meaningful than caring for an ill loved one?

Recovering a sense of purpose is, in a sense, a case of asking ourselves: 'what do I care about now?' If you don't know, don't worry. After a trauma, it often takes time and patience to re-discover what we care about. Just keep gently asking yourself – what do I care about? What inspires me? What matters to me? Look around and keep asking … what in the world calls me, what am I attracted to?

Having a purpose is what gets us out of bed in the morning. If it is a purpose that inspires us it will make it easier to get out of bed. If it is a purpose that is to merely keep us ticking over, there will be a greater temptation to snuggle back under the covers. Life is much more exciting when we care about and are inspired by what we do.

What would give *you* a meaningful life?

Remember that what gives you a meaningful life may not be the same for someone else and vice versa. There is no right or wrong. The world is made up of all sorts and that is what makes it such a wonder. Like an exotic fruit salad, if everyone wanted to be the banana, how boring and tasteless that would be.

You have the power to consciously create a meaningful life by asking:
What do I care about?
What moves me?
Where, in life, do I want to make a difference?

If you are unsure, gently keep asking … keep looking …

Once you have established an area of life where you wish to make a difference, you can begin to take steps that are consistent with what you are committed to in life.

For example: Let's say that Susie cares about animals. She wants to make a difference in the area of animal welfare. She wants to help protect animals from cruelty and help nurse injured animals back to health.

Her steps may look something like this.

1. Enquire at careers advisory service and universities or colleges about any courses in animal welfare. Veterinary nursing? Wildlife work?
2. Phone the local vet and ask if it may be possible to pop in for a quick chat for advice about working with animals.
3. Phone World Wildlife Trust – ask about opportunities for work either paid or voluntary for their organisation or other similar organisations.
4. Tell as many people as possible that she would like to work with animals. You never know, they may know someone who knows someone …
5. Through the internet, check out the animal rescue centres within the UK. Find out what sort of work they do in each one. How do they go about hiring people? Any job vacancies?
    Arrange to visit one for a weekend – volunteer services.
6. Phone the local riding school or boarding kennels. Tell them she is looking for experience working with animals. Could she go in once a week to help?
7. Phone the zoo and seek advice. How do people get to work with zoo animals? Have a list of questions to hand.

Living our purpose means putting our steps into action. Of course, there will be set-backs. Things will not go as we hope. Perhaps Susie gets an interview at college for veterinary nursing but doesn't get accepted on the course. This is not within her control. She can only do her best. The thing is don't give up, just re-commit to what you care about. Invent another step. Get work experience and apply next year. Keep going …

Purposes that involve other people thinking about us in a certain way can be dis-empowering. We cannot control what others think of us, we can only be responsible for ourselves.

Your purpose may change direction as you grow, develop. This is natural. The important thing is to be living your life in a way that gives your life meaning for you. A life that leaves you with a sense of satisfaction. If you don't know yet what that would be, don't worry...

Just keep looking, enquiring, exploring.

Recovering a Sense of Possibility

Your life for you
Breaking boundaries, creating a life you love.

You may feel it's now too late to do what you once wanted to do with your life … it's never too late.

Okay, let me clarify. Yes, there may be some things that you would have dearly loved to have done, that are now simply out of the equation. Perhaps in terms of having a child, from a purely biological point of view, this is no longer possible. You may have missed out on a profession that caters for younger people, like athletics or modelling. Perhaps you feel you lost the one man or woman you loved because of caring responsibilities.

There may be a sense of disappointment, sadness, perhaps anger that arises when you reflect on this. If so, this would be a good time to seek counselling to help you accept what has happened and the path that your life has followed thus far.

Problems arise when we can't accept the past. The past can weigh us down like lead, like poison. If all our regrets and 'failures' of the past live with us today, it can shut down our sense of what is possible for our life now, today and tomorrow.

When caring, a sense of possibility for your life was closed.

A sign read NO ENTRY. Now the sign reads OPEN!

Making choices about our lives when we are not used to it can feel terrifying. But we owe it to ourselves to ask: *Am I living a life I like?* What kind of life will I feel good about? What do I have to offer and, more importantly, enjoy doing?

You may feel that you have nothing to offer. Remind yourself of all your wonderful qualities. List them. Carers need courage, patience, compassion, stamina, boldness, strength, determination, reliability, organisational skills. The list goes on.

Accept the possibility that you did a wonderful, highly skilled job, that you are extremely talented and have a lot to offer not only the world, but yourself.

You may feel unsure about what you want to do. This is perfectly okay. Treat it as a game, an experiment. Many people do not know what they want to do in life.

Close your eyes and ask yourself, what do I really want for my life? Try to see yourself in pictures, images, rather than words. What are you doing? Where are you living? (I have included an exercise at the end that may help you establish some ideas).

Just because you have been a carer does not mean that you have to take the first job offered to you. Of course a lot will depend on your financial situation. When you are looking for work, try to identify a job that you might want to do, rather than being grateful for the first job that comes along. Value yourself and what you can offer. Making a conscious effort to find a job doing something that you want to do will give you a sense of self-esteem and fulfilment.

You may want to make an appointment to see a careers adviser. This service if free and often useful if you have been out of the job market for a long time. An advisor will direct you to the appropriate courses and give advice about grants or loans. There are also many associations that now offer free basic training for past carers in specific skills, your local carers centre would be able to tell you more.

Try out different things. Explore different avenues, mull over all your options. Keep asking yourself, is this what I really want to do with my life? Don't worry if you still have no clear idea, just keep exploring.

There is no such thing as a right or wrong decision, only a decision. If you make a choice to do something and it doesn't work out, then say to yourself 'Okay, I don't feel good about this, I'm going to do something else'.

There are no mistakes. There is only experience. Experience is how you find out.

If you are having trouble deciding what you want to do in your life, here are a couple of pointers that may help you.

Cast your mind back to when you were a child. Did the world seem full of possibilities? Did anything you want seem to be attainable? Remember when you used to say 'When I grow up I'm going to be a …' and it seemed absolutely within your reach to be that. Remember that feeling?

When I was about ten I wanted to join the circus. I wanted to stand on the back of the galloping, white horses, pink feathers bouncing between their ears, twisting in a sparkling leotard that danced golden beneath the spotlights. I wanted to cartwheel onto their backs and balance on one leg whilst waving to the crowd before I ascended a wire to the trapeze high above where I would effortlessly leap and swing, swing and leap. At the age of ten this seemed to be entirely possible, so logically possible that I had terrific trouble accepting my parents answer to my constant whine. "But why can't I join the circus?" (Answer) "You have to be born into it, they don't just take anyone." (Whine) "But I'm sure they'll accept ME. Can't we just at least try, can't we just at least ask them, pleeease?"

I have no doubt that, as an adult (had my performing desire not transformed into being an actress) – had I still harboured that burning desire to be in the circus, I could have taken steps to pursue that. Or at least I could have tried. It may not have worked out. I may have been more adept at landing under the horse than on it – but I would have had a go at something I wanted to do – and that is what counts.

Having A Go!

You owe it to yourself to have a go at what you really want to do in life. Often life interrupts our dreams, puts them on hold. They get so tired of waiting, they nod off, go to sleep. Be prepared that they are now lazy, cosy – they may take a wee time to stir. So wake them gently. Just a nudge here and there, little by little. Tell them it is safe to come out now. They have not been forgotten, only neglected.

Because of the incredible loss of confidence and self-esteem associated with long-term caring, we may feel afraid to re-awaken our dreams. What if it doesn't work out? The important thing is that you tried. And if things don't work out, there's always something else to try …

You may feel too exhausted to think about what you really want to do now. You may really not care what you do, it may seem too much effort. This is a natural part of grief. Just be with how you feel, never force anything until you are ready.

The point of this chapter is to simply help you be aware that there are avenues open to you that you may have believed were closed – you can make choices about what you want to do and the life you want to live – choices that help you realise your potential. Use every opportunity to seek out help from the appropriate government bodies or local groups that are there to help, encourage and support you. Don't be shy. Work with them in helping to establish what you want for your life. You deserve it.

EXERCISE

Sit or lie down in a comfortable position, cover yourself with a blanket, breathe deeply, inhaling energy from the air, exhaling any tension, relax the jaw. This is your time. You may like to play some quiet soothing music or perhaps ask a trusted friend or partner to read out the instructions. Or you may find it useful to tape the steps of the exercise first yourself, leaving enough time for a response.

Close your eyes. (Keep a pen and paper handy to jot down any images or memories afterwards.)

I invite you to cast your mind back to some happy memory of when you were a child.

Don't worry if nothing comes, just keep gently asking for a happy memory of childhood, somewhere between the ages of seven and twelve. Gently allow the memory to surface. In this memory, ask yourself a question. You can ask it aloud or to yourself. Ask this happy child 'What do you want to be when you grow up?' What is the response?

Now I invite you to remember a time in your life as a teenager, and recall a happy memory that you have between the ages of thirteen and eighteen. Ask this happy teenager 'Do you know what you'd like to do with your life?'

Don't force anything. If nothing comes this is absolutely okay, just enjoy the happy memory. If no happy memory comes, don't worry, be aware of lying or sitting in the room, be aware of your breath.

If you had clear responses to the question above (and they may possibly be different answers to the same question) I invite you to remember the feelings that accompanied the career or job that you had chosen. What sensations did the image of the career trigger in you? Excitement? Glamour? Respect?

Now move on to late teens, early adulthood. What did you actually do? Did you work? Were you unemployed? Studying? (this bit of the exercise will depend on how old you were when your caring role began). Visualise the images of you at work or in life before caring. If you were working, did you enjoy your job or was it something you just 'ended up' doing because other people expected that of you? Did you 'fall' into it because it was an easy option, or because you didn't know what else to do … or … gently let any answers arise, any sensations. If you had a few jobs before caring, then let various images surface. Try to identify the job you liked doing best of all.

Acknowledge and thank your memory for its hard work in this exercise. Now see yourself today, in this room, where you are sitting or lying. Get totally present to where you are now. Allow the images of the past to fade. Remember to breathe.

Now I invite you to imagine that you can have anything you want in life. Don't worry about how you would get it, just, for the purpose of this exercise, accept that you can have anything you wish, that this is an ideal world in which everything is possible. Try not to think too hard about the answers but rather enjoy this exercise as a visual treat, letting images float into your mind. Remember this is only a bit of fun and does not necessarily reflect your perfect life, but rather allows you to explore possibilities. It can be a useful tool to help us tune into any lost or new desires that perhaps we didn't even know existed.

I invite you to see yourself several years from now. It is a beautiful Spring day, the sun is shining. You are walking to work, the sun warm on your face. People smile as you arrive at work, they say 'good morning', ask you how you are doing, they are friendly and supportive.

You are doing a job you love, that gives you a great deal of satisfaction. You are good at your job. You enjoy getting up in the morning to come to work.

Where are you? What is your workplace like? Are you alone or working with others? What are you wearing? What are you doing? What are your particular responsibilities?

It has been another good day. The sun is still shining. It is time to go home. You say goodbye to the others. Someone asks you what you are doing that evening.

What do you tell them? What would your perfect evening look like? Are you alone or with others? What is your social life like?

See yourself carrying out your plans. Maybe you are going to a lovely restaurant with someone you love to eat dinner. Maybe you're going to play a sport or participate in a hobby. Maybe you're just going home to relax.

You have had a great evening and now you are home. This is your perfect house, not society's idea of a perfect house, but yours.

What is it like? How many rooms? What colour is the decoration? What is the furniture like? Where is your house? Town? Countryside? Abroad? Do you live alone or with others? Do you have any pets? Are you married? Boyfriend? Girlfriend? What are they like, what qualities draw you to them?

A friend calls. You share the great day you have had.

What do you tell her or him?

You arrange to meet this friend at the weekend.

What are you going to do? How often do you see your friends and family?

You go to bed.

What is your sex life like? What do you like to share intimately with your partner? With yourself?

You are in a lovely bed, cosy and warm. You fall into a deep, relaxed and easy sleep. You sleep right through until morning. You wake refreshed. The sun is streaming in. You make breakfast.

What do you eat? What is your ideal breakfast? What do you do before you leave for work?

You come out of the house into the sun. It is warm on your face. You are walking, people smile at you and nod as you pass them. You feel good, you are looking forward to the day ahead.

See yourself walking further away and wave goodbye. Thank yourself for allowing this insight into your perfect life. Gently let go of any images and allow yourself to become fully present to being here today sitting or lying in this room. Wriggle your toes, fingers, be aware of any sounds outside. Slowly open you eyes.

You may want to jot down or draw any pictures that came up for you.

Drink a couple of glasses of water to help cleanse the body.

Note

You can use the information you receive in this exercise to help establish a direction for your life. Then keep yourself open to the Universe and see if any opportunities come along that would support and encourage you to move forward in that direction. Often we miss those opportunities because we have not been able to really identify what we want. Your images or answers to questions in this exercise may change and vary depending on your mood and this is fine, natural. It is simply a fun way to get in touch with ourselves and perhaps unearth a way of being for our life that we had never been aware of before, had long forgotten or always thought impossible. Realise that you have choices and can create a life that you really want to, for you.

A new life.

Recovering a Sense of Strength

... in being vulnerable ...

Strength and vulnerability are two sides of the same coin. Both compliment the other. In allowing ourselves to be vulnerable in a healthy way, we allow ourselves to become stronger.

Asking for help is not a weakness but rather a valid way of helping yourself. It is a healthy recognition that we are not infallible but flesh and blood human beings.

Instead of struggling alone and sinking ever faster, we take responsibility for our welfare in asking for help. We ask from a position of choice, of power, rather than waiting until things get so bad that decisions either have to be taken out of our hands or we ask from a rock-bottom state. Before we get to that point we pick up the phone and say 'I need help'.

In acknowledging that we have been through a tough time, a traumatic time, in accepting that we are run-down and worn-out we pick up the phone and say 'I need help'.

In recent years the government has recognised the growing needs of carers. Many organisations have been specifically set up to provide help. In seeing that we are not 'bothering' those people but that they are (for the most part) paid a good wage, that they are doing their *job,* we see that it is perfectly reasonable to drop into one of these organisations and say 'I need help'. Many GP practices now offer counselling to their patients. You can ask your GP to refer you for counselling or direct you to an organisation that may be able to provide this service. It is up to you to ask. Tell people what you need. Only by telling people what we need will they know what to provide. People love to help. Sometimes they are just waiting to be asked.

I have listed below a number of organisations but seek out ones that are appropriate for you. (Your local library should have access to the internet if there is no postal address.) If there is currently no help available for what you need, be assertive. Find out who is in charge of the resources for your area and put your request in writing. It may be that this is an area, either geographically or emotionally, that they have never considered before. Being strong and asking for help could make a difference for someone else. Don't be shy …

Emotional support and carers organisations

If you are currently a carer, *Crossroads* provides support for carers to have a few hours off from their caring duties. To find out more contact the Crossroads (UK) on 01788 573653 or Northern Ireland 028 9181 4455 or visit www.crossroadscare.co.uk

Many Carers Organisations offer a free counselling service to current carers and past carers. Some also have information about Grants and Bursary schemes that are available to assist carers and past carers to re-train to improve work opportunities or simply to learn a new skill to build self-esteem and confidence. *The Princess Royal Trust for Carers* has two schemes available of this kind. Certain restrictions apply. All applications should be submitted through a Princess Royal Trust Carers centre. To find the centre closest to you, call The Princess Royal Trust for Carers Head Offices for (Scotland) 0141 221 5066 or (rest of UK) 020 7 480 7788. Or visit www.carers.org

Carers UK (formerly Carers National) offers information and support for carers. To find out what's available in your area call their Head Office on 020 7 490 8818 or visit www.carersonline.org.uk

The Alzheimer's Society may offer a support group for former carers of people with Dementia (depending on your area.) To find out more contact their Head Office on 020 7 306 0606 or call the Alzheimer's Helpline on 0845 3000 336

VOCAL (Voice Of Carers Across Lothian) are running a six-week course specifically for past carers called 'Letting Go, Moving On'. The course will explore various aspects of grief and loss of identity.

This is only available for carers in the Edinburgh area of Scotland. (If you think this kind of thing would be helpful to you, why not contact your local Carers Centre and ask if it may be possible to set something up in your area? Edinburgh carers can contact VOCAL on 0131 622 6666

For support with bereavement and grief, *CRUSE* is an organisation that helps to promote the well-being of bereaved people. For details of your local branch of Cruse call (Scotland) 01738 444 178 or (rest of UK) 020 8 939 9530

For bereaved parents or families who have lost a child (or children) *The Compassionate Friends* is a worldwide organisation that offers understanding and support. Contact their Helpline on 0117 953 9639 to find out what is available in your area.

Winston's Wish is a charity which supports bereaved children and young people. They also offer information and guidance to their families and to anyone concerned about a child after a bereavement. General enquiries: 01452 394377. Family Line: 0845 2030 405 (UK local rate).

The Way Foundation provides a self-help social and support network for men and women widowed under the age of 50, and their children. The main aim is to help those widowed young to rebuild their lives by helping one another. Telehone: 0870 011 3450 or write to The WAY Foundation, PO Box 74, Penarth, Cardiff CF64 5ZD or visit www.wayfoundation.org.uk

The Lesbian and Gay Bereavement Project offers support to bereaved gay men and lesbians, their families and friends. Call the Helpline (Mon–Fri 7pm–10.30pm) on 0207 403 5969

Samaritans – The Samaritans offer emotional support 24-hours a day. Call: 08457 90 90 90

Help the Aged Senior Line – advice and support for older people Telephone: 0808 800 6565

Communities

There are many communities throughout the world, each with their own ethos. Here I have listed the two I talk about in this book.

The *Bruderhof Community* publishes a number of books on death, dying and grief, exploring these issues from a Christian perspective. Call (freephone): 0800 018 0799 (The Darvell Bruderhof in East Sussex for more information)

For more information on *Thanantology, Music for the Dying*, call Judith Martin on 01479 811929 for information and workshops at the Findhorn Foundation call 01309 690311

Education

Learndirect is an organisation that helps people get back into learning but who may be unsure where to start – or simply need to talk to someone about the options available. There may also be help towards the costs of courses, particularly for those who are unemployed or on low-income. For more details about the funding options and courses available, call (Freephone) Learndirect 0800 100 9000 or 0800 101 901

To find out more about what courses are offered at your local *Further Education College* visit (for Scotland) www.2lc.info; (for England) www.bubl.ac.uk/uk/fe or (Northern Ireland) www.namss.org.uk

For other learning opportunities visit *The Open University* site at www.open.ac.uk

For people over the age of 50, who are no longer in gainful employment, the *University of the Third Age* offers courses in all sorts of subjects. It costs £10 per annum to join (£15 for a couple). To find out what is happening in your area contact The University of the Third Age, 26 Harrison Street, London WC1H 8JG. Telephone: 020 7 837 8845 or visit website www.u3a.org.uk

Social Life and Hobbies

For lone parents in England and Wales Gingerbread offers support. Call their advice line on (freephone) 0800 018 4318 open Monday to Friday 9–5pm. Or visit www.gingerbread.org.uk

If you are a single parent and wish to make contact and get support from others in a similar situation visit www.singlesparents.org

To meet people, and expand your social life, why not check out www.spiceuk.com. They say their main age group is in their 30s but they welcome people from all ages and backgrounds.

Natural Friends is an introduction agency for singles sharing interests in personal and spiritual growth. Call 0800 281 933.

Fancy a holiday but on your own? Why not check out *Solos,* who specifically cater for single people aged between 28-69. You can find out more on www.solosholidays.co.uk or call for a brochure 08700 – 746453. They are based at 54-58 High Street, Edgware, Middlesex HA8 7EJ.

If you are single and a Christian and wish to meet other single Christians visit www.christianconnection.co.uk (for Christians in the UK and Ireland).

Feel like you're in a rut? Why not check out www.latinnet.co.uk or www.letsdancesalsa.com to find out where Latin American dancing classes are in your area.

NB. There are numerous dating sites now on the internet but please do beware! Never go to someone's house but arrange to meet in a busy public place, and don't give out your address or phone number until you feel completely at ease.

Sex and Relationships

Relate offers counselling to adult couples with relationship difficulties, whether or not they are married. Telephone: (01788) 573241 or look in the phone book for your local centre.

The *Outsiders Trust* is a self-help group for people isolated because of a physical or social disability. It was set up to help people gain confidence by making friends and finding partners. Outsiders Trust is a registered charity. There are currently around 800 members. Membership is £22 (£11 unwaged) per calendar year. Further details from Outsiders Trust, PO Box 28724, London E18 1XW or call 0707 499 3527 (slightly more than local call rate) or visit www.outsiders.org.uk

If you are interested in finding out more about *Tantric Sex,* a company called *Transcendence* lists a wide variety of books on the subject. To find out more log on to www.martinj.dircon.co.uk

Alternative Therapies

Fancy yoga? Then visit www.yoga.co.uk to find out more.

If you are interested in finding out about alternative health care, (massage, reflexology, aromatherapy etc) then log on to the *British Register for Alternative Practice* site at www.brap.co.uk to find out what therapies are available in your area. Or call the British Complementary Medicine association on 0845 345 5977

Remember most Yellow Pages list many relevant self-help organizations.

Your local library will have a directory of useful numbers. Or surf the internet. Or phone your local council.

Speak up … ask for help … don't be shy

PAST CARING - The journey so far

When I first tried to get *Past Caring* published I was met with resistance from publishers. The replies were along the lines of "we like the idea but we are not confident a book on this subject would find a market." (Perhaps this goes some way towards explaining the lack of books available on caring for the seven million carers in the UK?) After countless rejections it seemed the only way to make the book happen was to publish it myself. I set up Promenade Publishing, took a mail-box, stored one thousand books in my bedroom, stuffed books into envelopes and dashed to and from the post office each day.

It was not long before *Past Caring* took on a life of its own. Readers wrote back to purchase more copies. They told me they had wanted to give *Past Caring* to a friend, their GP, their local hospice. Professional therapists and counsellors wrote to say how useful they had found the book in their work. A nurse told me reading *Past Caring* had made her change the way she related to the families of ill patients, showing them "much more compassion". *Past Caring* began to appear on university recommended reading lists for students of Social Work and Healthcare. A reader wrote to say he wanted to sponsor a copy to be sent to the Open University to be considered as reading for social science students. A minister from Cumbria sent me umpteen cheques explaining he kept "giving his own copy away. This is positive." One morning my e-mail flashed up a message from the University of Woolongong in New South Wales. A psychology professor there had read about *Past Caring* in the *Guardian* and wanted a copy for the university library. Carers groups leaders wrote to ask permission to photocopy sections of the book to use as handouts, to tell me they had been doing the exercises outlined in the recovery guide, to say reading *Past Caring* had inspired the setting up of a new past carers group. I received letters from centre mangers of The Princess Royal Trust for Carers saying how much their members had identified with the book and would I like to come and chat about it? (Although I was amazed at the PRT Centre Manager in Ayr who told me she "didn't have £8.99 in her budget to buy a copy of *Past Caring* for members to borrow!") I sent a copy of *Past Caring* to the Chief Executive of the NHS in Scotland which resulted in copies being distributed to healthcare professionals throughout Scotland in the hope of providing increased understanding and support for carers and past carers. A letter arrived from a man in Oban saying "I have never been a carer but I have been enthralled by *Past Caring* - or more honestly humbled by it. It has been like looking into a house through a window from the outside." A lady who was undergoing treatment for cancer wrote saying although she had never been a carer she identified with so many emotions in the book and had found it of invaluable help "at such a vulnerable time". And then there were the hundreds of letters from readers, current carers and past carers, who filled my mail-box to say 'thank you', to tell me how reading *Past Caring* had helped in their own healing and how *Past Caring* was the only source of comfort "I have found in the six months since my father died".

Past Caring was soon sold out.

I was amazed. Moved. Humbled. I was bloody thrilled. As well as branching out to past carers, *Past Caring* was making an impact at a grass roots level. New seeds of understanding were being planted. And who knows what this may mean for the carers and past carers of the future?

WHAT OTHERS SAY ABOUT PAST CARING

"Here is a book that those who long to begin living, after a career of caring, can identify with. This book will be of help to them as they seek out a suitable path for their new life. It is a giver of hope in what is often a truly devastating loss of purpose."

Dame Cicely Saunders, Founder of the Hospice Movement

"A great source of support and practical advice for many individuals who are feeling isolated and anxious about moving on."

Jo Ridley, MS Society

Extracts from letters:

"I have been unable to put the book down! I was gripped by the stories and emotions they evoked. I could readily identify with the issues you faced whilst caring and afterwards, from my personal experience of caring and that of carers I support through my work. Carers will take comfort from knowing how others deal with the overwhelming nature of caring and I believe the book gives sound advice on the subject of carers attending to their own needs. It will also help the bereaved carer regain confidence by recognising the valuable skills they have acquired through caring. Thank you again for such a valuable resource!

Jan Mussi, Carers Support Officer,
The Princess Royal Trust for Carers, Bristol and South Gloucs.

Thank you for writing *Past Caring*. It has been an enormous help to me - knowing my feelings and reactions are understandable and not unique has given me much needed courage to carry on. I found it difficult to take at first, emotions being stirred - but the way the book is written, in short narratives, meant I could put it down and pick it up again when I felt strong enough. I will be recommending it to other carers and I am buying two more copies. One will be to lend out (I don't want to lose my own copy) and the other will be for the Organisation 'Carers in Hertfordshire.' I just can't thank you enough.

(Mrs) Cathleen Palmer, Herts

I found *Past Caring* inspirational and was unable to put it down until I'd completed it. I had been a carer for over 25 years for my mother with Multiple Sclerosis. I felt that I couldn't continue and needed to make a break from caring. My mother is now in residential care, where she remains to this day. I felt bereaved in many ways and had difficulty in moving on - lots of feelings surrounding guilt, at no longer looking after my mother. Your book has been extremely beneficial in helping me move on and recognise that my feelings are normal and part of the process.

Zoe Nightingale, Wexford

When my mother died I simply kept going, partly to avoid the tremendous feeling of loss and partly because other people expected me to do so. When the surprising and overwhelming exhaustion finally hit me two years later, I didn't attribute it that much to the years of caring until I read your book and heard about other people's experiences. What a relief! I then saw that it was alright for me to simply stop and rest, it was alright for me to spend time caring for myself <u>and</u> it was alright to acknowledge to myself and to tell others that for 15 years I had had a *career* as a carer. I could give myself credit for choosing to do that. Thank you Audrey for helping me to own and understand my caring and past caring experience.

Kay Lee, Teddington

I read *Past Caring* from cover to cover in one sitting. I was given a copy by a friend who is a counsellor and she says she finds it very valuable in her counselling work. Long term caring has long term after effects and you have so eloquently identified the needs to be recognised. Thank you for bringing these issues to public recognition and also helping former carers take comfort in realising that they are not alone in the complexity of their situation. I'm off now to re-read your book and this time I'll try to put more of Part Three into practice!

Ros Nolan, Milton Keynes

Thanks!

So many people to thank. Like at a wedding I'm terrified I'll forget someone. Unlike Miss World this list is in no particular order.

I could never have done this book without the generosity of the carers. . . My heartfelt thanks to each and every one of you who took the time to meet me or write to me.
Thanks also to:
Jessie Bruce and Janis Silver for overseeing my Millennium Award; an angel Isobel Bruce who gave up her time for free to type the work I lost when my disc caught a virus; Julie Oswald and Lesley Warner who put me in touch with carers; my 'tea team' who fed and watered me (a starving artiste!) whilst I was writing - Marge, Dennis, Nicola, Tim, Brian, Aunty Doreen, Uncle James, Cousin Shona, Aunty Ena and Aunty Gladys, Kitchener's Deli, Jamieson's Cafe and Mr Hot Potato. Thank you Jennie Cowan for taking care of late-night faxes; Muttley Masters who came to the rescue as Transport Manager by supplying a new bike; the great writer Nicholas Mosley who encouraged me to write about my own life, and to dear friend Joanna Gibbs who has known me through it. Thanks to kind Jane Jeffrey who helped with Mum in the final days; Janet Bremner for the wonderful massages; Christeen Winford for providing a roof over my head, and Landmark Team - Chris, Tim, David, Dorrie, Heather and Stephen for coaching me on this journey through laughter and tears. Douglas S. Cutt for the fab photos; Suzanne Dance for the reading; Phil Rowlands and Helen Boden for the writing advice, and meditation group, Jamie, Mairi, Laura and Nathan and Punya for zapping me with loving energy. My eternal thanks to The Mingle Mania Nomad for working miracles; the overwhelming support of the Taylor family and to Indigo (PR) Ltd for donating their expertise. I am indebted to Isobel & Colin Leckie, David & Dorrie Bell and Kay Lee for helping spread the word. To the Broons, Anthony, Matthew, Sarah and Sophie, thanks for bringing fun to my life and (poet) Neil Bruno Broon for believing in me. Brian Rice, for his love, patience and constantly agreeing to tear himself away from the Comedy Channel to be a guinea pig for my 'listen-to-this-bit-and-this-bit-and-tell-me-what-you-prefer' testing. Big brother Haig and

sister Fiona, thanks for not saying (least not too often) what not finished yet? And to all those who worked so hard on the first edition, Liz Short, Andrew Simmons, Jim Hutcheson, Mark Blackadder, Kev, Charlie Tait, Amiten Palmer and Sam Wardle, without whose original efforts a second edition could not exist. I am grateful to those kind souls who sent donations towards the research for this book (p. 185), whose actions empowered me to take the first step at the bottom of the mountain - who took the risk that I might or might not make it to the top. And finally a huge thank you to ALL my friends who put up with me never returning their calls because I was writing, yet still called back to leave messages of love and support on my answer-phone, messages that kept me going and going and got me here. I thank you, my friends, with all my heart.